American Psychiatric Glossary

SEVENTH EDITION

Editorial Advisory Board

American Psychiatric Glossary

SEVENTH EDITION

Edited by

Jane E. Edgerton
Washington, D.C.

Robert J. Campbell III, M.D.
Editor, *Psychiatric News*
Director, Gracie Square Hospital
New York, New York

American
Psychiatric
Press, Inc.

Washington, DC
London, England

Copyright © 1994 American Psychiatric Press, Inc.

ALL RIGHTS RESERVED

Manufactured in the United States of America on acid-free paper

First Edition 97 96 95   4 3 2

American Psychiatric Press, Inc.
1400 K Street, N.W., Washington, DC 20005

Library of Congress Cataloging-in-Publication Data
American psychiatric glossary / edited by Jane E. Edgerton,
   Robert J. Campbell III. — 7th ed.
       p.   cm.
   Includes bibliographical references.
   ISBN 0-88048-526-4. — ISBN 0-88048-508-6 (pbk.)
   1. Psychiatry—Dictionaries. I. Edgerton, Jane E., 1945–   .
II. Campbell, Robert Jean, 1926–   .
RC437.S76 1994   94-5700
616.89′003—dc20   CIP

British Library Cataloguing in Publication Data
A CIP record is available from the British Library.

Contents

Dedication

This edition of the Glossary is dedicated to the memory of Evelyn Stone. As Director of Scientific Publications at McLean Hospital in Belmont, Massachusetts, she had a distinguished career as both editor and writer. She compiled and edited the sixth edition of the Glossary and served as a mentor to me and to others who strive to make the language of psychiatry understood and appreciated. Evelyn set a wonderful example.

Jane E. Edgerton

Introduction

The seventh edition of the *American Psychiatric Glossary* will help make the words used to outline and describe psychiatric disorders, symptoms, and situations involving the same easier to understand.

In any science, definitions of words must be modified to reflect new findings in research and current, updated information. This glossary reflects the momentous changes made in the diagnostic categories by the newly published fourth edition of the *Diagnostic and Statistical Manual of Mental Disorders* (DSM-IV). In addition, those terms from older nomenclatures that are used by and familiar to people who have not yet become acquainted with DSM-IV have been retained in this edition of the Glossary.

Those words appearing in italics within a definition are defined elsewhere in the glossary.

Many people made significant contributions to this book. Special thanks go to Ross Baldessarini, M.D., at McLean Hospital, Belmont, Massachusetts, for the "Table of Drugs Used in Psychiatry" and for definitions of drugs; Ralph Tarter, Ph.D., at Western Psychiatric Institute and Clinic's Center for Education and Drug Abuse Research, Pittsburgh, Pennsylvania, for updating the "Table of Psychological Tests"; Robert I. Simon, M.D., for the "List of Legal Terms"; Sheldon I. Miller, M.D., Chairman of Psychiatry and Behavioral Sciences at Northwestern University Medical School, Chicago, Illinois, for initial assistance with terms and concepts about addiction; and Michael First, M.D., Editor, DSM-IV text and criteria and New York State Psychiatric Institute, New York City, for making glossary definitions consistent with DSM-IV.

Others who wrote definitions and made suggestions about wording include Magda Campbell, M.D.; Joseph Carey, editor of the Society for Neuroscience's *Brain Facts* ; Sharon Cohen, American Psychiatric Association (APA) Government Relations; Gwenn Giedd, M.D.; Jay Giedd, M.D.; Corky Hart; Richard A. Isay, M.D.; Howard D. Kibel, M.D.; Ronald Martin, M.D.; Nicholas Meyers, APA Government Relations; Harold Alan Pincus, M.D.; Thomas J. Reckford; Steven S. Sharfstein, M.D.; James J. Strain, M.D.; Fred R. Volkmar, M.D.

Robert J. Campbell III, M.D., and I hope this glossary will help the reader to understand better the meanings of words encountered that have special meaning when used in the context of psychiatry.

Jane E. Edgerton

A

abnormality In psychological terms, any mental, emotional, or behavioral activity that deviates from culturally or scientifically accepted norms.

abreaction Emotional release or discharge after recalling a painful experience that has been repressed because it was not consciously tolerable (see *conscious*). A therapeutic effect sometimes occurs through partial or repeated discharge of the painful *affect*. See also *systematic desensitization*.

abstinence Foregoing some kind of gratification; in the area of alcohol or drug dependence, being without the substance on which the subject had been dependent.

abstract attitude (categorical attitude) A type of cognitive functioning that includes assuming a mental set voluntarily; shifting voluntarily from a specific aspect of a situation to the general; keeping in mind simultaneously various aspects of a situation; grasping the essentials of a whole, and breaking it into its parts and isolating them voluntarily; planning ahead ideationally; and/or thinking or performing symbolically. A characteristic of many psychiatric disorders is the person's inability to assume the abstract attitude or to shift readily from the concrete to the abstract and back again as demanded by circumstances.

abulia Lack of will or motivation, often expressed as inability to make decisions or set goals. See LIST OF NEUROLOGIC DEFICITS.

abuse (child, elder, spouse) To misuse, attack, or injure. The abuse may be sexual, physical, or emotional. See *abused child*.

abuse, substance Impairment in social and occupational functioning resulting from the pathological and "compulsive" use of a substance. The concept is closely related to the definition of substance dependence, which has similar *symptoms* of impairment but may include evidence of physiological *tolerance* or *withdrawal.* Typical symptoms of abuse include failure to fulfill major role obligations at work, school, or home; recurrent use of the substance in situations where such use is physically hazardous; substance-related legal problems; and continued use even though it causes or exaggerates interpersonal problems. See also *dependence, substance.*

abused child A child or infant who has suffered repeated injuries, which may include bone fractures, neurologic and psychological damage, or sexual abuse at the hands of a parent, parents, or parent surrogate(s). The abuse takes place repeatedly and is often precipitated, in the case of physical abuse, by the child's minor and normally irritating behavior. Child abuse also includes child neglect.

academic problem School difficulty that is not due to a *mental disorder.* Examples are failing grades or significant underachievement in a person with adequate intellectual capacity.

academic skills disorders In DSM-IV, this is a major group of *infancy, childhood, and adolescence disorders* that includes *reading disorder, mathematics disorder,* and disorder of *written expression.*

acalculia See LIST OF NEUROLOGIC DEFICITS.

accident-proneness Susceptibility to accidents based on psychological causes or motivations, usually *unconscious.*

accreditation Official certification that established standards have been met, such as the process by which hospitals and health facilities are surveyed and approved by the *Joint Commission on Accreditation of Healthcare Organizations (JCAHO).*

acculturation difficulty A problem in adapting to or finding an appropriate way to adapt to a different culture or environment. The problem is not based on any coexisting *mental disorder.*

acetylcholine A *neurotransmitter* in the brain, where it helps to regulate memory, and in the peripheral nervous system, where it controls the actions of skeletal and smooth muscle. See also *phobia.*

acting out Expressions of *unconscious* emotional conflicts or feelings in actions rather than words. The person is not consciously aware of the meaning of such acts (see *conscious*). Acting out may be harmful or, in controlled situations, therapeutic (e.g., children's play therapy).

actualization Realization of one's full potential.

acute confusional state 1) A form of *delirium* in which the most prominent *symptoms* are disorders of memory and orientation, usually with *short-term memory* deficit and both retrograde and anterograde *amnesia* and clouding of consciousness (i.e., reduced clarity of awareness of environment with reduced capacity to shift, focus, and sustain attention to environmental stimuli). See *organic mental disorder.* 2) An acute stress reaction to new surroundings or new demands, common in *adolescence;* it generally subsides as the person adjusts to the situation. See also *identity crisis.*

adaptation Fitting one's behavior to meet the needs of one's environment, which often involves a modification of impulses, emotions, or attitudes.

adiadochokinesia See LIST OF NEUROLOGIC DEFICITS.

addiction Dependence on a chemical substance to the extent that a physiological and/or psychological need is established. This may be manifested by any combination of the following symptoms: tolerance, preoccupation with obtaining and using the substance, use of the substance despite anticipation of probable adverse consequences, repeated efforts to cut down or control substance use, and *withdrawal symptoms* when the substance is unavailable or not used.

ADHD See *attention-deficit/hyperactivity disorder.*

adjustment Often transitory functional alteration or accommodation by which one can better adapt oneself to the immediate environment and to one's inner self. See also *adaptation.*

adjustment disorder An imprecise term referring to emotional or behavioral *symptoms* that develop in response to an identifiable stressor. The symptoms, which may include *anxiety,* depressed mood, and disturbance of conduct, are clinically significant in that the distress exceeds what would be expected under the circumstances, or significant impairment in social or occupational functioning is produced. Duration of symptoms tends to be self-limited, not persisting more than 6 months after termination of the stressor or its consequences. Sometimes the disorder is designated as "acute" if duration is 6 months or less, and as "persistent" or "chronic" if symptoms endure beyond 6 months.

Adler, Alfred (1870–1937) Viennese *psychiatrist,* founder of the school of *individual psychology.* See also *compensation; masculine protest; overcompensation.*

administrative psychiatry The branch of psychiatry that deals with the organization of clinical practice in a program, hospital, or other facility. Its focus is on the management process involving interaction of health administration; clinical care of psychiatric patients; and the attitudes, values, and belief systems of the organization.

adolescence A chronological period of accelerated physical and emotional growth leading to sexual and psychological maturity. It often begins at about age 12 and ends at a loosely defined time, when the individual achieves independence and social productivity (usually about age 20). See also *psychosocial development; psychosexual development.*

adolescent psychiatry See *child and adolescent psychiatry.*

adrenergic Referring to neural activation by *catecholamines* such as *epinephrine, norepinephrine,* and *dopamine.* See also *biogenic amines; neurotransmitter; sympathetic nervous system.*

adrenergic system That system of organs and nerves in which *catecholamines* are the *neurotransmitters.*

advance directive See *living will.*

adverse effects See *side effect.*

affect Behavior that expresses a subjectively experienced feeling state (*emotion*); affect is responsive to changing emotional states, whereas mood refers to a pervasive and sustained emotion. Common affects are euphoria, anger, and sadness. Some types of affect disturbance are:

> **blunted** Severe reduction in the intensity of affective expression.

> **flat** Absence or near absence of any signs of affective expression such as a monotonous voice and an immobile face.

> **inappropriate** Discordance of voice and movements with the content of the person's speech or ideation.

> **labile** Abnormal variability, with repeated, rapid, and abrupt shifts in affective expression.

> **restricted or constricted** Reduction in the expressive range and intensity of affects.

affective disorder A disorder in which mood change or disturbance is the primary manifestation. Now referred to as *mood disorder.* See *depression.*

aftercare Posthospitalization program of rehabilitation designed to reinforce the effects of therapy and to help the patient adjust to his or her environment and prevent relapse.

age-associated memory impairment (AAMI) The mild disturbance in memory function that occurs normally with aging; benign senescent forgetfulness.

aggression Forceful physical, verbal, or symbolic action. May be appropriate and self-protective, including healthy self-assertiveness, or inappropriate as in hostile or destructive behavior. May also be directed toward the environment, toward another person or *personality,* or toward the self, as in *depression.*

aging Characteristic pattern of life changes that occur normally in humans, plants, and animals as they grow older. Some age changes begin at birth and continue until death; other changes begin at maturity and end at death.

agism Systematic stereotyping of and discrimination against elderly people. It is distinguished from gerontophobia, a specific pathological fear of old people and aging.

agitated depression A severe major depressive disorder in which *psychomotor agitation* is prominent; formerly known as *involutional melancholia.* See *depression.*

agitation Excessive motor activity, usually nonpurposeful and associated with internal tension. Examples include inability to sit still, fidgeting, pacing, wringing of hands, and pulling of clothes. See *psychomotor agitation.*

agnosia Failure to recognize or identify objects despite intact sensory function; may be seen in *dementia.* See LIST OF NEUROLOGIC DEFICITS.

agonist In pharmacology, a substance that stimulates or mimics a receptor-mediated biological response by occupying cell receptors. Contrast to *antagonist.*

agoraphobia *Anxiety* about being in places or situations in which escape might be difficut or embarrassing or in which help may not be available should a *panic attack* occur. The fears typically relate to venturing into the open, of leaving the familiar setting of one's home, or of being in a crowd, standing in line, or traveling in a car or train. Although agoraphobia usually occurs as a part of *panic disorder,* agoraphobia without a history of panic disorder has been described.

AIDS Acquired immune deficiency syndrome; a cluster of disorders such as Kaposi's sarcoma (KS) and opportunistic infections to which the subject is abnormally vulnerable because of collapse of the immune defense system. The cause is a retrovirus, human T-lymphotropic virus type III (HTLV-III) or HIV (human immunodeficiency virus), which infects and suppresses the T4 lymphocyte, the focal cell of the immune system. It also directly attacks specific types of cells in the *central nervous system* (CNS) and lungs (and perhaps in other tissues as well). There is no known cure, and the mortality rate is high.

Over 40% of AIDS patients develop neurologic complications at some point in their illness. The most common CNS dysfunction is a generalized encephalopathy or progressive multifocal leukoencephalopathy (PML) that includes *dementia* as a dominant feature. Less commonly, the dysfunction is due to well-defined focal lesions, including opportunistic infection by Toxoplasma gondii, which may invade nervous tissue and give rise to seizures or more subtle alterations in mentation and behavior. Cases with a presenting picture of acute *psychosis* without dementia have also been described. Myelopathy and peripheral neuropathy are other neurologic complications.

AIDS dementia complex See *HIV dementia.*

ailurophobia See *phobia.*

akathisia, neuroleptic-induced, acute Complaints of restlessness accompanied by movements such as fidgeting of the legs, rocking from foot to foot, pacing, or inability to sit or stand. *Symptoms* develop within a few weeks of starting or raising the dose of a *neuroleptic* medication or of reducing the dose of medication used to treat extrapyramidal symptoms (see *extrapyramidal syndrome*).

akinesia A state of motor inhibition; reduced voluntary movement. See also LIST OF NEUROLOGIC DEFICITS.

akinetic mutism See LIST OF NEUROLOGIC DEFICITS.

Al-Anon A 12-step program for relatives of alcoholic persons operating in many communities under the philosophical and organizational structure of *Alcoholics Anonymous* to facilitate discussion and resolution of common problems.

Alateen A 12-step program for teenage children of alcoholic parents operating in some communities under the philosophical and organizational structure of *Alcoholics Anonymous*. Alateen provides a setting in which the children may receive group support in achieving an understanding of their parents' problems and in learning better methods of coping.

alcohol amnestic disorder (Korsakoff's syndrome) A disease associated with chronic alcoholism and resulting from a deficiency of vitamin B_1. Patients sustain damage to part of the thalamus and cerebellum and have anterograde and retrograde *amnesia,* with an inability to retain new information. In alcohol amnestic disorder, unlike *dementia,* other intellectual functions may be preserved. See also *alcohol psychosis; Wernicke-Korsakoff syndrome.*

alcohol dependence Dependence on alcohol characterized by either tolerance to the agent or development of *withdrawal* phenomena on cessation of, or reduction in, intake. Other aspects of the syndrome are psychological dependence and impairment in social and/or vocational functioning. This is also called alcoholism.

Alcohol, Drug Abuse, and Mental Health Adminis-tration (ADAMHA) An agency in the U.S. Department of Health and Human Services that was replaced in 1992 by the Substance Abuse and Mental Health Services Administration (SAMHSA). In reorganizing ADAMHA into SAMHSA, the three ADAMHA research institutes, the National Institute on Alcohol Abuse and Alcoholism (NIAAA), the National Institute on Drug Abuse (NIDA), and the National Institute of Mental Health (NIMH), were moved to the *National Institutes of Health*. What remain in SAMHSA are the substance abuse and mental health services programs.

alcohol hallucinosis An *organic mental disorder* consisting of auditory *hallucinations* occurring in a clear *sensorium,* developing shortly after the reduction or cessation of drinking, usually within 48 hours. The disorder commonly follows prolonged and heavy alcohol use.

alcohol psychosis A group of major *mental disorders* associated with organic brain dysfunction due to alcohol; in DSM-IV, categorized as alcohol-induced psychotic disorder. Includes *delirium tremens* and *alcohol hallucinosis.*

alcohol use disorders In DSM-IV, this group includes alcohol dependence, alcohol abuse, alcohol intoxication, alcohol withdrawal, alcohol delirium, alcohol persisting dementia, alcohol persisting amnestic disorder, alcohol psychotic disorder, alcohol mood disorder, alcohol anxiety disorder, alcohol sleep disorder, and alcohol sexual dysfunction. See *abuse, substance; dependence, substance; intoxication, alcohol; withdrawal symptoms, alcohol.*

alcohol withdrawal syndrome See *withdrawal symptoms, alcohol.*

Alcoholics Anonymous (AA) A 12-step program for alcoholic persons who collectively assist other alcoholic persons through a structured fellowship of personal and group support. See also *Al-Anon; Alateen.*

alcoholism   See *alcohol dependence.*

Alexander, Franz (1891–1964)   Hungarian-born *psychoanalyst* who was a professor of *psychiatry* at the University of Chicago; his chief contributions were in the areas of brief analysis and *psychosomatic* medicine.

alexia   Loss of the ability to grasp the meaning of written or printed words and sentences. See LIST OF NEUROLOGIC DEFICITS. See also *dyslexia.*

alexithymia   A disturbance in affective and cognitive function that overlaps diagnostic entities but is common in *psychosomatic disorders,* addictive disorders, and *posttraumatic stress disorder.* The chief manifestations are difficulty in describing or recognizing one's own emotions, a limited fantasy life, and general constriction in the affective life.

algophobia   Fear of pain. See *phobia.*

alienation   The estrangement felt in a setting one views as foreign, unpredictable, or unacceptable. For example, in *depersonalization* phenomena, feelings of unreality or strangeness produce a sense of alienation from one's self or environment. In *obsessions,* which involve a fear of one's emotions, avoidance of situations that arouse emotions, and continuing effort to keep feelings out of awareness, there is alienation of *affect.*

alienist   Obsolete term for a *psychiatrist* who testifies in court about a person's sanity or mental competence.

allied health professional   A member of a nonmedical profession whose functions traditionally include involvement in the prevention, treatment, or rehabilitation process. In *psychiatry,* examples include the *psychiatric nurse, psychiatric social worker,* clinical *psychologist,* neuropsychologist, occupational therapist, and art therapist.

alloplastic   Referring to *adaptation* by means of altering the external environment. Contrast to *autoplastic,* which refers to the alteration of one's own behavior and responses.

alogia   Literally, speechlessness. Most commonly used to refer to the lack of spontaneity in speech and diminished flow of conversation that occur as *negative symptoms* in *schizophrenia.*

alter ego transference   See *transference, selfobject.*

alveolar hypoventilation syndrome   *Sleep apnea.* See *breathing-related sleep disorder.*

Alzheimer's disease   A progressive, increasing impairment in memory and other intellectual functions/activities beginning with confusion and forgetfulness. The progression, usually after 1 to 2 years, is shown in disorientation, muscle rigidity, purposeless hyperactivity, and difficulty in speaking. The final stage shows the patient with *dementia* and in a vegetative state. See *senile dementia.*

The dementia is characterized by continuing and gradual cognitive and functional decline. Early-onset type (sometimes called *presenile dementia*) occurs at age 65 or younger; late-onset type occurs after the age of 65. In the course of deterioration, various syndromes may be superimposed such as *depression, delusions, hallucinations,* or other perceptual, behavioral (violence), communication, or motor skill disturbances.

ambivalence   The coexistence of contradictory emotions, attitudes, ideas, or desires with respect to a particular person, object, or situation. Ordinarily, the ambivalence is not fully *conscious* and suggests psychopathology only when present in an extreme form.

amentia   Subnormal development of the mind, with particular reference to intellectual capacities; a type of severe *mental retardation.*

American Board of Psychiatry and Neurology, Inc. (ABPN) A group of 16 physicians that arranges, controls, and conducts examinations to determine the competence of specialists in *psychiatry,* child psychiatry, *neurology,* and neurology with special competence in child neurology. The group consists of 5 physicians from the *American Psychiatric Association,* 4 from the American Neurological Association, 3 from the Section Council on Psychiatry of the American Medical Association, 2 from the American Academy of Neurology, and 2 from the Section Council on Neurology of the American Medical Association. Recently, it established examinations for added qualifications in geropsychiatry and addiction psychiatry.

American Journal of Psychiatry The official monthly scientific publication of the *American Psychiatric Association.*

American Law Institute formulation See under *insanity defense* in LIST OF LEGAL TERMS.

American Psychiatric Association (APA) The leading national professional organization in the United States for physicians who specialize in *psychiatry.* Members are from the United States, Canada, Central America, and the Caribbean Islands, and corresponding members are from other countries. Founded in 1844 as the Association of Medical Superintendents of American Institutions for the Insane, the Association changed its name to the American Medico-Psychological Association in 1891 and adopted its present name in 1921. The Association is governed by a board of 21 elected trustees whose primary function is to formulate and implement the policies and programs of the Association, and by an Assembly of District Branches representing the membership. Numerous councils, committees, commissions, and task forces furnish the data and recommendations on which the Trustees and Assembly base their deliberations. The Association had more than 37,700 members in 1993. Its headquarters are at 1400 K Street, N.W., Washington, D.C. 20005.

amimia A disorder of language characterized by an inability to make gestures or to understand the significance of gestures. See also *learning disability; speech disturbance.*

amines Organic compounds containing the amino group (–NH2); of special importance in biochemistry and neurochemistry because of their role as *neurotransmitters. Epinephrine* and *norepinephrine* are amines. See also *biogenic amines.*

amino acids Any organic acid containing one or more amino (–NH2) groups. The *biogenic amines* (among which are *dopamine, epinephrine, norepinephrine,* and *serotonin*) are of particular importance in neurochemistry because of their role as *neurotransmitters.*

amnesia Pathologic loss of memory; a phenomenon in which an area of experience becomes inaccessible to *conscious* recall. The loss in memory may be organic, emotional, dissociative, or of mixed origin, and may be permanent or limited to a sharply circumscribed period of time. Two types are distinguished:

anterograde Inability to form new memories for events following such a condition(s).

retrograde Loss of memory for events preceding the amnesia proper and the condition(s) presumed to be responsible for it.

amnestic disorder A cognitive disorder characterized by impairment of memory that is manifested in an inability to learn new information and to recall previously learned knowledge. It is termed transient if impairment lasts for 1 month or less or persistent if impairment lasts more than 1 month. Amnestic disorder may be substance induced (in particular alcohol and sedative/hypnotic/anxiolytic drugs) or due to a general medical condition (including physical trauma).

amok See *culture-specific syndromes.*

amphetamine use disorders In DSM-IV, this group includes amphetamine (or related substance) dependence, amphetamine abuse, amphetamine intoxication, amphetamine withdrawal, amphetamine delirium, amphetamine psychotic disorder, amphetamine mood disorder, amphetamine anxiety disorder, amphetamine sexual dysfunction, and amphetamine sleep disorder.

amphetamines A group of chemicals that stimulate *dopamine* release in the *central nervous system;* often misused by adults and adolescents to control normal fatigue and to induce *euphoria.* Used clinically to treat *hyperkinetic disorder* and *narcolepsy.*

amygdala In the structure of the brain, part of the *basal ganglia* located on the roof of the temporal horn of the lateral ventricle at the inferior end of the caudate nucleus. It is a structure in the forebrain that is an important component of the limbic system.

amyloid Any one of various complex proteins that are deposited in tissues in different disease processes. These proteins have an affinity for Congo red dye. In *neuropsychiatry,* of particular interest are the beta-amyloid (A4) protein, which is the major component of the characteristic senile *plaques* of *Alzheimer's disease,* and the amyloid precursor protein (APP).

amyotrophic lateral sclerosis Motor *neuron* disease of unknown etiology characterized by progressive degeneration of corticospinal tracts and anterior horn cells or bulbar efferent neurons. Commonly known as "Lou Gehrig's disease." *Symptoms* are progressive and include wasting of the upper limbs, then of the tongue, larnyx, and pharynx; difficulty in speech (*dysarthria*); painful swallowing (*dysphagia*); and death in 1 to 4 years.

anaclitic Literally, leaning on. In psychoanalytic terminology (see *psychoanalysis*), dependence of the infant
on the mother or mother substitute for a sense of
well-being. Normal behavior in childhood, but pathologic in later years.

anal character A *personality* type that manifests excessive orderliness, miserliness, and obstinacy. Called
obsessive-compulsive character or personality in other
typologies. In *psychoanalysis,* a pattern of behavior in
an adult that is believed to originate in the *anal
phase* of infancy, between 1 and 3 years. See also
psychosexual development.

anal phase See *psychosexual development.*

analgesia Absence of appreciation of painful sensations.

analysand A patient in psychoanalytic treatment (see
psychoanalysis).

analysis A common synonym for *psychoanalysis.*

analytic psychology The name given by the Swiss
psychoanalyst Carl Gustav *Jung* to his theoretical
system, which minimizes the influences of sexual
factors in emotional disorders and stresses mystical
and religious influences and a belief in the collective
unconscious. See also *anima; persona.*

anamnesis The developmental history of a patient and
of his or her illness, especially recollections.

anankastic personality Synonym for obsessive-
compulsive personality. See *obsessive-compulsive*
under *personality disorder.*

ancillary care Health services other than professional
services or hospital room and board; these services
may include drug and laboratory services.

androgyny A combination of male and female characteristics in one person.

anesthesia Absence of sensation; may result from
nerve damage, anesthetic drugs, or psychological

processes such as in *hysterical neurosis, conversion type* (see under *neurosis*) or *hypnosis*.

anhedonia Inability to experience pleasure from activities that usually produce pleasurable feelings. Contrast with *hedonism*.

anima In Jungian psychology, a person's inner being as opposed to the character or *persona* presented to the world. Further, the anima may be the more feminine "soul" or inner self of a man, and the animus the more masculine soul of a woman. See also *Jung*.

anniversary reaction An emotional response to a previous event occurring at the same time of year. Often the event involved a loss and the reaction involves a *depressed* state. The reaction can range from mild to severe and may occur at any time after the event.

anomie Apathy, alienation, and personal distress resulting from the loss of goals previously valued. Emile Durkheim popularized this term when he listed it as a principal reason for *suicide*.

anorexia nervosa An *eating disorder* characterized by refusal or inability to maintain minimum normal weight for age and height combined with intense fear of gaining weight, denial of the seriousness of current low weight, undue influence of body weight or shape on self-evaluation, and, in females, amenorrhea or failure to menstruate. Weight is typically 15% or more below normal, and it may decrease to life-threatening extremes. In the restricting subtype, the person does not engage regularly in binge eating. In the binge eating/purging, or bulimic, subtype, the person engages in recurrent episodes of *binge eating* or purging during the episode of anorexia nervosa. See also *bulimia nervosa*.

anorgasmia The inability to achieve *orgasm*. See *orgasm disorders*.

anosognosia See LIST OF NEUROLOGIC DEFICITS.

Antabuse (disulfiram) A drug used in treatment of *alcohol dependence* to create an aversive response to alcohol. It blocks the normal metabolism of alcohol and produces increased blood concentrations of acetaldehyde that induce distressing *symptoms* such as flushing of the skin, pounding of the heart, shortness of breath, nausea, and vomiting. With more severe reactions, hypotension, cardiovascular collapse, and, sometimes, convulsions may occur.

antagonist In pharmacology, a substance that opposes, blocks, or neutralizes a receptor-mediated biologic response. For example, the morphine antagonist *naloxone* competes with morphine for receptor sites in the brain and other tissues. By occupying these sites, naloxone prevents the narcotic from binding to the receptors and exerting its effect. Contrast with *agonist*.

antianxiety drugs See TABLE OF DRUGS USED IN PSYCHIATRY.

anticholinergic effects or properties Interference with the action of *acetylcholine* in the brain and peripheral nervous systems by any drug. In *psychiatry,* the term generally refers to the side effects of *antipsychotic drugs, tricyclic antidepressants,* and *antiparkinsonian drugs.* Common symptoms of such effects include dry mouth, blurred vision, and constipation.

antidepressant drugs See TABLE OF DRUGS USED IN PSYCHIATRY.

antimanic drugs See TABLE OF DRUGS USED IN PSYCHIATRY.

antiparkinsonian drugs Pharmacologic agents that ameliorate Parkinson-like *symptoms.* In *psychiatry,* these agents are used to combat the untoward Parkinson-like and extrapyramidal effects (see *extrapyramidal syndrome*) that may be associated with treatment with phenothiazines and other antipsychotic drugs.

antipsychotic drugs See TABLE OF DRUGS USED IN PSYCHIATRY.

antisocial behavior Conduct indicating indifference to another's person or property; criminal behavior, dishonesty, or abuse are examples. In DSM-IV, childhood or adolescent antisocial behavior and adult antisocial behavior (in contrast to antisocial personality disorder, etc.) are included as "other conditions that may be a focus of clinical attention."

antisocial personality See *personality disorder.*

anxiety Apprehension, tension, or uneasiness from anticipation of danger, the source of which is largely unknown or unrecognized. Primarily of *intrapsychic* origin, in distinction to *fear,* which is the emotional response to a consciously recognized and usually external threat or danger. May be regarded as pathologic when it interferes with effectiveness in living, achievement of desired goals or satisfaction, or reasonable emotional comfort.

anxiety disorders In DSM-IV, this category includes panic disorder without agoraphobia, panic disorder with agoraphobia, agoraphobia without history of panic disorder, specific (simple) phobia, social phobia (social anxiety disorder), obsessive-compulsive disorder, posttraumatic stress disorder, acute stress disorder, generalized anxiety disorder (includes overanxious disorder of childhood), anxiety disorder due to a general medical condition, and substance-induced anxiety disorder. (The inclusion of mixed anxiety-depressive disorder into this category awaits further study.) See *agoraphobia; generalized anxiety disorder; mixed anxiety-depressive disorder; obsessive-compulsive disorder; panic disorder; phobia; posttraumatic stress disorder.*

anxiety hysteria An early psychoanalytic term (see *psychoanalysis*) for what is now called *phobia.*

anxiety neurosis See under *neurosis.*

anxiety-depressive disorder, mixed See *mixed anxiety-depressive disorder.*

anxiolytics Drugs that have an antianxiety effect and are used widely to relieve emotional tension. The most commonly used antianxiety drugs are the *benzodiazepines.* See TABLE OF DRUGS USED IN PSYCHIATRY.

apathy Lack of feeling, emotion, interest, or concern.

aphasia Loss of the ability to use or understand words; may be seen in *dementia.* See LIST OF NEUROLOGIC DEFICITS.

aphonia Inability to produce normal speech sounds; may be due to either organic or psychological causes.

apoplexy See *stroke.*

apperception Perception as modified and enhanced by one's own *emotions,* memories, and biases.

apraxia Inability to carry out motor activities despite intact comprehension and motor function; may be seen in *dementia.* See LIST OF NEUROLOGIC DEFICITS.

ARC *AIDS*-related complex; a group of *symptoms* that appear to represent premonitory signs of full-blown AIDS, such as generalized lymphadenopathy (disease involving the lymph nodes), night sweats, persistent fevers, persistent cough, infection of the throat, and prolonged diarrhea.

arithmetic disorder See *mathematics disorder.*

arousal disorder, autonomic See *autonomic arousal disorder.*

arousal disorder, sexual See *sexual arousal disorders.*

arteriosclerosis See *cerebral arteriosclerosis.*

articulation disorder See *phonological disorder.*

artificial intelligence (AI) A computer using ideas and methods of computation; investigators use AI to understand and recreate the principles that make intelligence possible.

Asperger's disorder A disorder of development characterized by gross and sustained impairment in social interaction and restricted, repetitive, and stereotyped patterns of behavior, interests, and activities occurring in the context of preserved cognitive and language development.

assertiveness training A procedure in which subjects are taught appropriate interpersonal responses involving frank, honest, and direct expression of their feelings, both positive and negative.

assimilation A Piagetian term (see *Piaget*) describing a person's ability to comprehend and integrate new experiences.

association Relationship between ideas and *emotions* by contiguity, continuity, or similarity. See also *free association; mental status*.

astereognosis See List of Neurologic Deficits.

ataxia Loss of muscle coordination; irregularity of muscle action. See List of Neurologic Deficits.

attachment The behavior of an organism that relates in an affiliative or dependent manner to another object. This attachment develops during critical periods of life and can be extinguished by lack of opportunity to relate. If this separation occurs before maturation can provide for adaptive adjustment, personality deviation can occur. See *bonding*.

attachment disorder, reactive A disorder of infancy or early childhood, beginning before the child is 5 years old, characterized by markedly disturbed and developmentally inappropriate social relatedness. In the inhibited type of reactive attachment disorder, failure to respond predominates, and responses are hypervigilant, avoidant, or highly ambivalent and contradictory. *Frozen watchfulness* may be present. In the disinhibited type, indiscriminate sociability is characteristic, such as excessive familiarity with relative strangers or lack of selectivity in choice of attachment figures. The majority of children who develop this disorder (either type) are from a setting in which care has been grossly pathogenic. Either the caregivers have continually disregarded the child's basic physical and emotional needs, or repeated changes of the primary caregiver have prevented the formation of stable attachments.

attachment learning The theory that the presence of someone to whom one is emotionally attached has a special effect on how one learns, especially in infancy.

attention Ability to sustain focus on one activity. A disturbance in attention may appear as having difficulty in finishing tasks that have been started, being easily distracted, or having difficulty in concentrating.

attention-deficit/hyperactivity disorder (ADHD) A child whose inattention and hyperactivity-impulsivity cause problems may have this disorder. *Symptoms* appear before the age of 7 years and are inconsistent with the subject's developmental level and severe enough to impair social or academic functioning.

In the predominantly inattentive type, characteristic symptoms include distractibility, difficulty in sustaining attention or following through on instructions in the absence of close supervision, avoidance of tasks that require sustained mental effort, failure to pay close attention to details in schoolwork or other activities, difficulty in organizing activities, not listening to what is being said to him or her, loss of things that are necessary for assignments, and forgetfulness in daily activities.

In the predominantly hyperactive-impulsive type, characteristic symptoms are that the person inappropriately leaves his or her seat in classroom or runs about, fidgets or squirms, has difficulty in engaging in leisure activities quietly, has difficulty in awaiting turn in games, and blurts out answers to questions before they are completed.

The two types may be combined.

atypical An adjective used to describe unusual or un-characteristic variations of a disorder.

atypical depression In DSM-IV, depressive *symptoms* that do not meet the criteria for specific depressive disorders. See also *depression.*

atypical psychosis In DSM-IV, a psychotic disorder not otherwise specified; a residual category for the occurrence of psychotic symptoms that do not meet the criteria for a specific psychotic disorder. See also *psychosis.*

audit (medical audit, patient care audit) Periodic and systematic review of patterns of patient care to assess the quality of treatment.

aura A premonitory, subjective brief sensation (e.g., a flash of light) that warns of an impending headache or convulsion. The nature of the sensation depends on the brain area in which the attack begins. Seen in *migraine* and *epilepsy.*

authority figure A person in a position of power (e.g., a parent or parent surrogate).

autism A form of thinking or a style of object relation-ships and life approach in which the subjective pre-dominates and the "me" is favored, sometimes resulting in the exclusion of the "not-me." The subject is unable to turn his or her energies to outside reality. *Introversion* may be marked, with an avoidance of contact with life and satisfying relationships with peers.

autistic disorder A disorder of development consisting of gross and sustained impairment in social interaction and communication; restricted and stereotyped pat-terns of behavior, interest, and activities; and abnormal development prior to age 3 manifested by delays or abnormal functioning in social development, language communication, or play. Specific *symptoms* may in-clude impaired awareness of others, lack of social or emotional reciprocity, failure to develop peer relationships appropriate to developmental level, delay or absence of spoken language and abnormal nonverbal communication, stereotyped and repetitive language, idiosyncratic language, impaired imaginative play, insistence on sameness (e.g., nonfunctional routines or rituals), and stereotyped and repetitive motor mannerisms.

autistic fantasy Substitution of excessive daydreaming for the pursuit of relationships with others, for more direct and effective action, or for solving problems.

autoeroticism Sensual self-gratification. Characteristic of, but not limited to, an early stage of emotional development. Includes satisfactions derived from genital play, masturbation, fantasy, and oral, anal, and visual sources.

automatism Automatic and apparently undirected nonpurposeful behavior that is not consciously controlled. Seen in psychomotor *epilepsy.*

autonomic arousal disorder A disorder characterized by persistent or recurrent *symptoms* other than pain that are mediated by the *autonomic nervous system* and not a part of a *general medical condition.* Symptoms may involve various systems or organs including palpitations (cardiovascular), hyperventilation (respiratory), vomiting (gastrointestinal), urinary frequency (urogenital), or flushing (dermal). In earlier classifications (DSM-I, DSM-II, and DSM-III), such symptoms were considered conversion symptoms, psychosomatic symptoms, or psychophysiological disorders.

autonomic nervous system (ANS) The part of the nervous system that innervates the cardiovascular, digestive, reproductive, and respiratory organs. It operates outside of consciousness and controls basic life-sustaining functions such as heart rate, digestion, and breathing. It includes the *sympathetic nervous system* and the *parasympathetic nervous system.*

autoplastic Referring to *adaptation* by changing the self.

autopsy, psychological See *psychological autopsy.*

aversion disorder, sexual See *sexual desire disorders.*

aversion therapy A *behavior therapy* procedure in which stimuli associated with undesirable behavior are paired with a painful or unpleasant stimulus, resulting in the suppression of the undesirable behavior.

avoidant disorder Social *phobia* occurring in childhood and adolescence.

avoidant personality disorder See *personality disorder.*

avolition Lack of initiative or goals; one of the *negative symptoms* of *schizophrenia.* The person may wish to do something, but the desire is without power or energy.

axon The fiber-like extension of a *neuron* through which the cell sends information to target cells.

B

bad object One of the results of *splitting* of the psychic representations of objects into their pleasurable, exciting, good, supportive, nurturing, and needs-meeting aspects (i.e., the good object), and their unpleasurable, frustrating, undesirable, painful, deprecatory, damaged, critical, hostile, incomplete, and disavowed aspects (i.e., the bad object). Splitting is a normal *ego* mechanism during infantile development; in the adult it is a manifestation of an inability to integrate positive and negative qualities of the object (or self) into a cohesive image.

barbiturates Drugs that depress the activities of the *central nervous system;* primarily used for sedation or treatment of convulsive disorders. See TABLE OF DRUGS USED IN PSYCHIATRY.

basal ganglia Clusters of *neurons* located deep in the brain; they include the caudate nucleus and the putamen (corpus striatum), the globus pallidus, the subthalamic nucleus, and the substantia nigra. The basal ganglia appear to be involved in higher-order aspects of motor control, such as planning and execution of complex motor activity and the speed of movements.

Lesions of the basal ganglia produce various types of involuntary movements such as athetosis, chorea, *dystonia,* and *tremor.* The basal ganglia are involved also in the pathophysiology of *Parkinson's disease, Huntington's disease,* and *tardive dyskinesia.*

The internal capsule, containing all the fibers that ascend to or descend from the cortex, runs through the basal ganglia and separates them from the *thalamus.*

basic benefits In insurance policies, the minimum set of benefits that must be made available to the insured.

basic trust The infant's sense of security in his or her relationship with the mother (parents, caregiver) that makes it possible for the infant to begin to recognize the parent as other and separate from the self. It is the basis of *reality testing,* the ability to relate to others, and the feeling of self-worth and self-esteem.

battered child See *abused child.*

BEAM See *brain electrical activity mapping.*

Beers, Clifford W. (1876–1943) Author of *A Mind That Found Itself* and founder, in 1909, of the National Committee for Mental Hygiene, now the *National Mental Health Association.*

behavior disorders of childhood See *attention-deficit/hyperactivity disorder; disruptive behavior disorder.*

behavior modification See *behavior therapy*.

behavior therapy A mode of treatment that focuses on modifying observable and, at least in principle, quantifiable behavior by means of systematic manipulation of the environment and variables thought to be functionally related to the behavior. Some behavior therapy techniques are *operant conditioning, shaping, token economy, systematic desensitization, aversion therapy,* and *flooding (implosion)*. See also *biofeedback*.

behavioral neurology The branch of *neurology* that concerns itself with functioning, such as language, memory, and purposeful or motivated activity or *affect*.

behavioral sciences The study of human development, values, and interpersonal relations. The behavioral sciences encompass such fields as *psychiatry, psychology, cultural anthropology, sociology,* and political science.

behaviorism An approach to *psychology* first developed by *John B. Watson* that rejected the notion of mental states and reduced all psychological phenomena to neural, muscular, and glandular responses. Contemporary behaviorism emphasizes the study of observable responses but is directed toward general behavior rather than discrete acts. It includes private events such as feelings and *fantasies* to the extent that these can be directly observed and measured.

benzodiazepines The generic name for a group of drugs that have potent hypnotic, sedative, and anxiolytic action. They are also called *anxiolytics* or *antianxiety drugs*. See TABLE OF DRUGS USED IN PSYCHIATRY.

bereavement Feelings of deprivation, desolation, and grief at the loss of a loved one. The grieving person does not need to seek professional help unless these feelings last for a long period of time or relief is sought for *symptoms* such as *anorexia nervosa* or *insomnia*.

bestiality *Zoophilia;* sexual relations between a human being and an animal. See also *paraphilia*.

beta-blocker An agent that inhibits the action of beta-adrenergic receptors, which modulate cardiac functions, respiratory functions, and the dilation of blood vessels. Beta-blockers are of value in the treatment of hypertension, cardiac arrhythmias, and *migraine*. In *psychiatry,* they have been used in the treatment of aggression and violence, *anxiety*-related tremors and lithium-induced tremors, neuroleptic-induced *akathisia,* social phobias, panic states, and alcohol withdrawal.

binge drinking A pattern of heavy alcoholic intake that occurs in bouts of a day or more that are set aside for drinking. During periods between bouts, the subject may abstain from alcohol.

binge eating A period of time of overeating during which a larger amount of food is ingested than most people would eat during that time. The person feels that he or she cannot stop eating or has no control over what or how much is consumed. During the episode, the person may eat more rapidly than usual, eat until feeling uncomfortably full, eat large amounts of food although not feeling hungry, and eat alone because of embarrassment over how much is being eaten. After a bout of overeating, *depression,* guilt feelings, and feelings of disgust with oneself are common. When binge eating is accompanied by compensatory behavior to control weight, it is termed *bulimia nervosa*.

biochemistry The chemistry of living organisms and of the changes occurring therein.

bioenergetic psychotherapy See *experiential therapy*.

biofeedback The use of instrumentation to provide information (i.e., feedback) about variations in one or more of the subject's own physiological processes not ordinarily perceived (e.g., brain wave activity, muscle tension, blood pressure). Such feedback over a period of time can help the subject learn to control certain physiological processes even though he or she is unable to articulate how the learning was achieved.

biogenic amine hypothesis The concept that abnormalities in the physiology and metabolism of biogenic amines, particularly *catecholamines* (*norepinephrine* and *dopamine*) and an *indoleamine* (*serotonin*), are involved in the causes and courses of certain psychiatric illnesses. The concept was derived originally from a serendipitous discovery that *monoamine oxidase inhibitors* and certain tricyclic drugs had mood-elevating properties, and that these agents exerted dramatic effects on brain monoamine functions. The findings that *phenothiazines* and other *neuroleptics* inhibit dopamine activity in the brain further support this theory and suggest that a disorder of dopamine metabolism may be implicated in the etiology of *psychosis* or of *mania*. Also, disorders in norepinephrine and serotonin activity have been implicated in the etiology of *depression* and mania.

biogenic amines Organic substances of interest because of their possible role in brain functioning; subdivided into *catecholamines* (e.g., *epinephrine, dopamine, norepinephrine*) and *indoleamines* (e.g., tryptophan, *serotonin*). The biosynthetic pathway for the catecholamines is tyrosine → dihydroxyphenylalanine → dopamine → norepinephrine → epinephrine. The biosynthetic pathway for the indoleamines is tryptophan → serotonin (5-hydroxytryptamine) → 5-hydroxyindoleacetic acid (5-HIAA).

biological psychiatry A school of psychiatric thought that emphasizes physical, chemical, and neurologic causes of psychiatric illness and treatment approaches. See also OUTLINE OF SCHOOLS OF PSYCHIATRY.

biological rhythms Cyclical variations in physiological and biochemical function, level of activity, and emotional state. Circadian rhythms have a cycle of about 24 hours; ultradian rhythms have a cycle that is shorter than 1 day; and infradian rhythms have a cycle that may last weeks or months.

bipolar disorders In DSM-IV, a group of *mood disorders* that includes bipolar disorder, single episode; bipolar disorder, recurrent; and *cyclothymic disorder*.

A bipolar disorder includes a *manic* episode at some time during its course. In any particular patient, the bipolar disorder may take the form of a single manic episode (rare), or it may consist of recurrent episodes that are either manic or depressive in nature (but at least one must have been predominantly manic).

Bipolar II disorder is used in some classifications (including DSM-IV) to denote a mood disorder characterized by episodes of major depressive disorder and *hypomania* (rather than full mania). Other authorities prefer to call such a mood disorder "major depressive disorder with hypomanic episodes." See *hypomanic episode*.

bipolar self In the *self psychology* of Heinz *Kohut,* the final psychic structure that emerges following successful development and transformations of infantile constellations (equivalent to the mature human psyche of *id, ego,* and *superego*). The structure begins as the *nuclear self* made up of the *grandiose self* and the *idealized parental imago*. In successful development the grandiose self is transformed into self-assertive ambitions at one pole of the bipolar self. At the other pole are the internalized values and ideals that have grown out of the idealized parental imago. Between the two poles are the person's innate talents and skills.

birth trauma Term used by Otto *Rank* to relate his theories of *anxiety* and *neurosis* to what he believed to be the inevitable psychic shock of being born.

bisexuality Originally a concept of *Freud,* indicating a belief that components of both sexes could be found in each person. Today the term is often used to refer to persons who are capable of achieving *orgasm* with a partner of either sex. See also *gender role; homosexuality.*

Bleuler, Eugen (1857–1939) Swiss *psychiatrist* whose investigations of *dementia praecox* led him to outline a modern concept of *schizophrenia.*

blind spot Visual scotoma, a circumscribed area of blindness or impaired vision in the visual field; by extension, an area of the personality of which the subject is unaware, typically because recognition of this area would cause painful emotions.

blocking A sudden obstruction or interruption in spontaneous flow of thinking or speaking, perceived as an absence or deprivation of thought.

blood levels The concentration of a drug in the plasma, serum, or blood. In *psychiatry,* the term is most often applied to levels of *lithium carbonate, tricyclic antidepressants,* and anticonvulsants. Maximum clinical responses to these agents have been correlated with specific ranges of blood levels. See also *therapeutic window.*

blood-brain barrier The barrier (boundary) that excludes many molecules and substances from freely diffusing or being transported into the brain tissues from the blood stream; serves a protective function.

blunted affect See *affect.*

board-certified psychiatrist A *psychiatrist* who has passed examinations administered by the *American Board of Psychiatry and Neurology, Inc.,* and thus becomes certified as a medical specialist in *psychiatry.*

body dysmorphic disorder (BDD) One of the *somatoform disorders,* characterized by preoccupation with some imagined defect in appearance not of delusional intensity but severe enough to impair social or occupational functioning.

body image One's sense of the self and one's body.

body language The expression of feelings or thoughts transmitted by one's motions, posture, or facial expressions that have meaning within the context in which they appear. See also *kinesics.*

bondage See *masochism, sexual.*

bonding The unity of two people whose identities are significantly affected by their mutual interactions. Bonding often refers to the *attachment* between a mother and her child.

borderline See *personality disorder.*

borderline intellectual functioning An "additional condition that may be a focus of clinical attention" (DSM-IV), especially when it coexists with a disorder such as *schizophrenia.* The IQ is in the range of 71 to 84.

borderline personality disorder See *personality disorder.*

bradykinesia Neurologic condition characterized by a generalized slowness of motor activity.

brain The part of the nervous system confined in the skull; it includes the cerebrum, midbrain, cerebellum, pons, and medulla.

brain disorders See *organic mental disorder.*

brain electrical activity mapping (BEAM) Computer-enhanced analysis and display of electroencephalographic and evoked response studies. In evoked response studies, a stimulus (e.g., flashing light) is presented to the patient and the responses are recorded electrically from scalp electrodes. Computers translate the information into a topographic, colored display of electrical activity over the surface of the brain. Useful in diagnosing seizure disorders and helpful in looking at atypical psychiatric disorders. See also *brain imaging.*

brain imaging Any technique that permits the in vivo visualization of the substance of the *central nervous system.* The best known of such techniques is *computed tomography* (CT). Newer methods of brain imaging such as *positron-emission tomography* (PET) and *magnetic resonance imaging* (MRI) are based on different physical principles but also yield a series of two-dimensional images (or "slices") of brain regions of interest.

A number of other related techniques, such as ultrasound, SPECT (single-photon emission tomography), angiography in its various forms, regional cerebral blood flow (rCBF) measurements, *brain electrical activity mapping* (BEAM) and its variants, and even the older pneumoencephalogram (PEG), also provide images of some aspect of the central nervous system. However, these techniques are generally more invasive or limited in the structures visualized, the degree of resolution, or some other parameter, than CT, PET, SPECT, and MRI.

brain metabolism The process by which the brain synthesizes, degrades, and alters chemical substrates for repair and function.

brain stem The pons and the medulla oblongata. The major route by which the forebrain sends information to and receives information from the spinal cord and peripheral nerves. The brain stem controls, among other things, respiration and heart rhythms.

brain syndrome See *organic mental disorder.*

brain waves See *electroencephalogram.*

Brawner decision See *American Law Institute/Model Penal Code test* under *insanity defense* in LIST OF LEGAL TERMS.

breathing-related sleep disorder A *dyssomnia* characterized by sleep disruption that produces excessive sleepiness or *insomnia*. The disruption is due to *sleep apnea* or central alveolar hypoventilation syndrome.

brief depressive disorder See *depressive disorders*.

brief psychotherapy Any form of *psychotherapy* whose end point is defined either in terms of the number of sessions (generally not more than 15) or in terms of specified objectives; usually goal-oriented, circumscribed, active, focused, and directed toward a specific problem or *symptom*.

brief reactive psychosis See *psychotic disorder, brief*.

Brigham, Amariah (1798–1849) One of the original 13 founders of the *American Psychiatric Association* (1844) and the founder and first editor of its official journal, now the *American Journal of Psychiatry*.

Briquet's syndrome See *somatization disorder*.

bruxism Grinding of the teeth, occurs unconsciously while awake or during stage 2 *sleep*. May be secondary to *anxiety*, tension, or dental problems.

bulimia nervosa An *eating disorder* characterized by recurrent episodes of *binge eating* followed by compensatory behavior such as purging (i.e., self-induced vomiting or the use of diuretics and laxatives) or other methods to control weight (e.g., strict dieting, fasting, or vigorous exercise).

burnout A stress reaction developing in persons working in an area of unrelenting occupational demands. *Symptoms* include impaired work performance, fatigue, *insomnia, depression,* increased susceptibility to physical illness, and reliance on alcohol or other drugs of abuse for temporary relief.

buspirone An *anxiolytic* agent that is not related chemically to other antianxiety or hypnotic-sedative drugs and does not demonstrate *cross-tolerance* to them.

butyrophenones See TABLE OF DRUGS USED IN PSYCHIATRY.

C

caffeine use disorders In DSM-IV, this group includes caffeine intoxication, caffeine anxiety disorder, and caffeine sleep disorder.

cannabis See TABLE OF COMMONLY ABUSED DRUGS.

cannabis use disorders In DSM-IV, this group includes cannabis dependence, cannabis abuse, cannabis intoxication, cannabis delirium, cannabis psychotic disorder with delusions or hallucinations, and cannabis anxiety disorder.

Capgras' syndrome The delusion that others, or the self, have been replaced by imposters. It typically follows the development of negative feelings toward the other person that the subject cannot accept and attributes, instead, to the imposter. The *syndrome* has been reported in paranoid schizophrenia (see *schizophrenia*) and, even more frequently, in organic brain disease.

capitation A uniform fee or tax based on the number of people in the population being served. The health care provider, or group of providers, accepts responsibility to deliver the health services needed by all members of a specified group, and an agreed-upon payment is made at regular intervals to them. The payment is made even if no services have been given, but the payment is no greater than the agreed-upon amount even if very many services have been provided.

caregiver Any person involved in the treatment or rehabilitation of a patient; includes the *psychiatrist* and other members of the traditional treatment team as well as community workers and other nonprofessionals.

case management 1) A type of health care delivery with emphasis on the development of alternative treatment plans for the patients who have been identified (by preadmission certification, diagnosis, etc.) as potential high-cost cases. Once such a case has been identified, the case manager confers with the patient's physician to develop a less expensive treatment plan and aftercare. 2) The process of following a patient through various types of treatment and helping with care.

castration Removal of the sex organs. In psychological terms, the fantasized loss of the genitals. Also used figuratively to denote state of *impotence,* powerlessness, helplessness, or defeat.

castration anxiety *Anxiety* due to fantasized danger or injuries to the genitals and/or body. It may be precipitated by everyday events that have symbolic significance and appear to be threatening, such as loss of a job, loss of a tooth, or an experience of ridicule or humiliation.

catalepsy A generalized condition of diminished responsiveness shown by trancelike states, posturing, or maintenance of physical attitudes for a prolonged period of time. May occur in organic or psychological disorders, or under *hypnosis.*

cataplexy Sudden loss of postural tone without loss of consciousness, typically triggered by some emotional stimulus such as laughter, anger, or excitement. It is a characteristic of *narcolepsy.*

catatonia Immobility with muscular rigidity or inflexibility and at times excitability. See also *schizophrenia.*

catatonic behavior Marked motor abnormalities, generally limited to those occurring as part of a nonorganic psychotic disorder. This term includes catatonic *excitement* (apparently purposeless agitation not influenced by external stimuli), *stupor* (decreased reactivity and fewer spontaneous movements, often with apparent unawareness of the surroundings), *negativism* (apparent motiveless resistance to instructions or attempts to be moved), *posturing* (the person's assuming and maintaining an inappropriate or bizarre stance), *rigidity* (the person's maintaining a stance or posture against all efforts to be moved), and waxy flexibility, or *cerea flexibilitas* (the person's limbs can be put into positions that are maintained).

catatonic disorder due to general medical condition Secondary or symptomatic catatonia; catatonic *symptoms* such as motoric immobility (e.g., *catalepsy, cerea flexibilitas*), extreme agitation, extreme *negativism* (e.g., rigidity of posture), and peculiarities of voluntary movement (e.g., inappropriate or bizarre posturing, stereotyped movements, prominent mannerisms) that occur in relation to a *general medical condition*. This diagnosis emphasizes that catatonic symptoms are not confined to schizophrenic disorders.

catchment area A geographic area for which a mental health program or facility has responsibility for its residents.

catecholamines A group of *biogenic amines* derived from tyrosine and containing the catechol (3,y-di-hydroxyphenyl) moiety. Certain of these amines, such as *epinephrine, norepinephrine,* and *dopamine,* are *neurotransmitters* and exert an important influence on peripheral and *central nervous system* activity. See also *biogenic amine hypothesis.*

categorical attitude See *abstract attitude.*

catharsis The healthful (therapeutic) release of ideas through "talking out" *conscious* material accompanied by an appropriate emotional reaction. Also, the release into awareness of repressed ("forgotten") material from the *unconscious.* See also *repression.*

cathexis Attachment, *conscious* or *unconscious,* of emotional feeling and significance to an idea, an object, or, most commonly, a person.

causalgia A sensation of intense pain of either organic or psychological origin. See *somatoform disorders*.

central alveolar hypoventilation syndrome See *breathing-related sleep disorder; sleep apnea*.

central nervous system (CNS) The brain and the spinal cord.

cephalalgia Headache or head pain.

cerea flexibilitas The "waxy flexibility" often present in catatonic *schizophrenia* in which the patient's arm or leg remains in the position in which it is placed.

cerebral arteriosclerosis Hardening of the arteries of the brain sometimes resulting in an *organic mental disorder* that may be either primarily neurologic (e.g., convulsions, *aphasia,* chorea, athetosis, *parkinsonism,* etc.) or primarily psychological (e.g., intellectual dulling, memory deficits, emotional lability (see *affect*), paranoid *delusions,* and confusion), or a combination of both. In DSM-IV, it is termed *vascular dementia*.

cerebrovascular accident (CVA) See *stroke*.

character The sum of a person's relatively fixed *personality* traits and habitual modes of response.

character analysis Psychoanalytic treatment (see *psychoanalysis*) aimed at the *character defenses*.

character defense Any personality trait that serves an *unconscious* defensive purpose. See *defense mechanism*.

character disorder (character neurosis) A *personality disorder* manifested by a chronic, habitual, maladaptive pattern of reaction that is relatively inflexible, limits the optimal use of potentialities, and often provokes the responses from the environment that the person wants to avoid. In contrast to symptoms of *neurosis,* character traits are typically *ego-syntonic*. See also *personality*.

chemical dependence A generic term for dependence (addiction) on alcohol or other drugs. See *dependence, substance*.

child abuse See *abused child*.

child analysis Application of modified psychoanalytic methods (see *psychoanalysis*) and goals to problems of children to remove impediments to normal personality development.

child and adolescent psychiatry The diagnosis, prevention, and treatment of *mental disorders* in persons under the age of 18.

childhood disintegrative disorder See *disintegrative disorder*.

childhood schizophrenia See *schizophrenia*.

chlorpromazine See TABLE OF DRUGS USED IN PSYCHIATRY.

cholinergic Activated or transmitted by *acetylcholine* (e.g., parasympathetic nerve fibers). See also *parasympathetic nervous system*. Contrast with *adrenergic*.

cholinergic hypothesis The theory that the basic defect in *Alzheimer's disease* is an inadequacy of *acetylcholine* for neurotransmission.

chromosome 21 The chromosome involved in *Down syndrome* (21 trisomy), which is most frequently due to nondisjunction of chromosome 21, resulting in 3, rather than 2, chromosomes (and making the total 47 chromosomes, rather than the normal total of 46). In 1987 it was reported that the genetic defect in familial *Alzheimer's disease* is located on chromosome 21, the same chromosome of which there is an extra copy in Down syndrome. This supports the idea that at least one form of Alzheimer's is inherited and that a similar genetic defect may occur in both Down and familial Alzheimer's disorders.

chromosomes Microscopic, intranuclear structures that carry the *genes*. The normal human cell contains 46 chromosomes, consisting of 23 pairs of chromosomes—22 pairs of autosomes and 1 pair of sex chromosomes.

chronic Continuing over a long period of time or recurring frequently. Chronic conditions often begin inconspicuously, and *symptoms* may be less pronounced than in acute conditions.

chronobiology The science or study of temporal factors in life stages and disorders, such as the sleep-wake cycle, biological clocks and rhythms, and so forth.

circadian rhythms See *biological rhythms.*

circadian rhythm sleep disorder Sleep-wake schedule disorder; a *dyssomnia* consisting of sleep disruption leading to excessive sleepiness or *insomnia* that is due to a mismatch between the sleep-wake schedule required by a person's environment and his or her circadian sleep-wake pattern. In the delayed sleep phase type, sleep onset and awakening times are late and the person is unable to fall asleep and awaken at a desired earlier time. The desynchronized type includes sleep disruption produced by jet lag and by recurrent changes in work shifts; it is characterized by insomnia during the major sleep period or excessive sleepiness during the major wake period.

circumstantiality Pattern of speech that is indirect and delayed in reaching its goal because of excessive or irrelevant detail or parenthetical remarks. The speaker does not lose the point, as is characteristic of *loosening of associations,* and clauses remain logically connected, but to the listener it seems that the end will never be reached. Compare with *tangentiality.*

clanging A type of thinking in which the sound of a word, rather than its meaning, gives the direction to subsequent associations. Punning and rhyming may substitute for logic, and language may become increasingly a senseless *compulsion* to associate and decreasingly a vehicle for communication. For example, in response to the statement "That will probably remain a mystery," a patient said, "History is one of my strong points."

claustrophobia See *phobia*.

climacteric Menopausal period in women. Sometimes used to refer to the corresponding age period in men. Also called involutional period.

clinical psychologist See *psychologist*.

clinical social worker A social worker who applies the theory and methods of social work to the treatment and prevention of psychosocial dysfunction, disability, or impairment with individuals, families, and small groups. Many states require a license to practice clinical social work. Usually certification requires a master's degree in social work, at least 2 years' work experience, and the passing of an examination. See *social work*.

clouding of consciousness See *acute confusional state*.

clozapine See TABLE OF DRUGS USED IN PSYCHIATRY.

cluster suicides Multiple *suicides,* usually among adolescents, in a circumscribed period of time and area. Thought to have an element of contagion.

CME See *continuing medical education*.

coactive strategy The use of more than one drug to achieve a desired response. Combination is the use of two or more drugs with different mechanisms of action but the same response. Augmentation is the addition of one or more drugs to enhance the effects of the drug(s) already being used.

cocaine A naturally occurring stimulant drug found in the leaves of the coca plant, Erythroxylon coca. Its systemic effects include nervous system stimulation, manifested by garrulousness, restlessness, excitement, delusional ideas, a false feeling of increased strength and mental capacity, and epileptic seizures.

cocaine use disorders In DSM-IV, this group includes cocaine dependence, cocaine abuse, cocaine intoxication, cocaine withdrawal, cocaine delirium, cocaine psychotic disorder with delusions or hallucinations, cocaine mood disorder, cocaine anxiety disorder, cocaine sexual dysfunction, and cocaine sleep disorder.

codependency A popular term referring to all the effects that people who are dependent on alcohol or other substances have on those around them, including the attempts of those people to affect the dependent person. The term implies that codependence is a psychiatric disorder and hypothesizes that the family's actions tend to perpetuate (enable) the person's dependence. Empirical studies, however, support a stress and coping model for explanation of the family behavior.

cognition A general term encompassing all the various modes of knowing and reasoning.

cognitive Refers to the mental process of comprehension, judgment, memory, and reasoning, in contrast to emotional and volitional processes. Contrast with *conative*.

cognitive development Beginning in infancy, the acquisition of intelligence, *conscious* thought, and problem-solving abilities. An orderly sequence in the increase in knowledge derived from sensorimotor activity has been empirically demonstrated by *Piaget*. See also *psychosexual development; psychosocial development*.

cognitive disorders In DSM-IV, this group includes *delirium, dementia,* and *amnestic disorder*.

cognitive-behaviorial psychotherapy Cognitive therapy; a short-term psychotherapy directed at specific target conditions or *symptoms*. (*Depression* has been the most intensively investigated to date.) The symptoms themselves are clues to the patient's verbal thoughts, images, and assumptions that account for both the symptomatic state and the psychological vulnerability to that state. Initial treatment is aimed at symptom reduction. The patient is taught to recognize the negative cognitions that contribute significantly to the development or maintenance of symptoms and to evaluate and modify such thinking patterns. The second phase of treatment concerns the underlying problem.

cognitive-emotional therapies See *experiential therapy.*

cohesive self The stable sense of one's *identity* or core self, which develops through progressive consolidation of the grandiose self, the idealized parental *imago,* and the person's talents and skills. Optimal development is promoted by a *holding environment* in which the child develops *basic trust.*

collective unconscious In Jungian theory, a portion of the unconscious common to all people; also called "racial unconscious." See also *analytic psychology; Jung; unconscious.*

coma A severe disturbance of consciousness with absence of voluntary activity and diminished or absent responsiveness to tactile, thermal, proprioceptive, visual, auditory, olfactory, or verbal stimuli. Coma is indicative of widespread cerebral dysfunction and is often part of *delirium.*

combat fatigue An outmoded term for *posttraumatic stress disorder.* Disabling physical and emotional reaction incident to military combat. Paradoxically, the reaction may not necessarily include fatigue.

commitment A legal process for admitting, ordinarily involuntarily, a mentally ill person to a psychiatric treatment program. The legal definition and procedure vary from state to state, although commitment usually requires a court or judicial procedure. Commitment may also be voluntary.

communication disorders In DSM-IV, this group includes expressive language disorder, mixed receptive/expressive language disorder, *phonological disorder,* and *stuttering.*

In developmental expressive language disorder, scores on tests measuring expressive language development are below those on tests of nonverbal intelligence and those on tests measuring receptive language. *Symptoms* may include limited vocabulary, speaking only in the present tense, errors in recalling words, and developmentally inappropriate sentence length.

Mixed receptive/expressive language disorder is characterized by testing performance on both receptive and expressive language development batteries that is substantially below performance on nonverbal intellectual batteries. The typical manifestation is an inability to understand words or sentences. (Pure receptive language disorder is not seen; receptive disorders are always accompanied by expressive language deficits.)

community mental health center (CMHC) A mental health service delivery system first authorized by the federal Community Mental Health Centers Act of 1963 to provide a comprehensive program of mental health care to *catchment area* residents. The CMHC is typically a community facility or a network of affiliated agencies that serves as a locus for the delivery of the various services included in the concept of *community psychiatry.*

community psychiatry That branch of *psychiatry* concerned with the provision and delivery of a coordinated program of mental health care to residents of a geographic area. These efforts include working with patients, their families, and agencies within the community. Goals are the prevention of mental illness as well as care and treatment for those persons with *mental disorders.*

comorbidity The simultaneous appearance of two or more illnesses, such as the co-occurrence of *schizophrenia* and substance abuse or of *alcohol dependence* and *depression*. The association may reflect a causal relationship between one disorder and another or an underlying vulnerability to both disorders. Also, the appearance of the illnesses may be unrelated to any common *etiology* or vulnerability.

compensation A *defense mechanism,* operating unconsciously (see *unconscious*), by which one attempts to make up for real or fancied deficiencies. Also a *conscious* process in which one strives to make up for real or imagined defects of physique, performance skills, or psychological attributes. The two types frequently merge. See also *Adler; individual psychology; overcompensation.*

compensation neurosis Factitious or artificial illness complicated by unresolved monetary claims. See *secondary gain.*

competency to stand trial See LIST OF LEGAL TERMS.

complex A group of associated ideas having a common, strong emotional tone. These ideas are largely *unconscious* and significantly influence attitudes and associations. See also *Oedipus complex.*

compulsion Repetitive ritualistic behavior such as hand washing or ordering or a mental act such as praying or repeating words silently that aims to prevent or reduce distress or prevent some dreaded event or situation. The person feels driven to perform such actions in response to an *obsession* or according to rules that must be applied rigidly, even though the behaviors are recognized to be excessive or unreasonable.

compulsive Refers to intensity or repetitiveness of behavior rather than to compulsive behavior strictly defined. Thus, "compulsive drinking" and "compulsive gambling" refer to cravings that may be intense and often repeated, but they are not viewed as compulsions.

compulsive personality See *personality disorder.*

computed tomography (CT) A technique for imaging anatomic structures using X ray. Objects are exposed to a series of X-ray beams on a single plane but with origin at different points around a 180-degree arc. A computer algorithm reconstructs the beam absorption data so as to display an image of absorption values at each point in the plane. The process is repeated for each plane to be imaged. Used for anatomic abnormalities such as strokes, tumor, and atrophy of the brain. See also *brain imaging.*

computerized axial tomography (CAT) scanning See *computed tomography (CT).*

conative Pertains to one's basic strivings as expressed in behavior and actions; volitional as contrasted with *cognitive.*

concordance See LIST OF RESEARCH TERMS.

concrete thinking Thinking characterized by immediate experience, rather than abstractions. It may occur as a primary, developmental defect, or it may develop secondary to organic brain disease or *schizophrenia.*

concussion An impairment of *brain* function caused by injury to the head. The speed and degree of recovery depend on severity of the brain injury. *Symptoms* may include headache, disorientation, paralysis, and unconsciousness.

condensation A psychological process, often present in dreams, in which two or more concepts are fused so that a single symbol represents the multiple components.

conditioning Establishing new behavior as a result of psychological modifications of responses to stimuli.

conditioning, operant See *operant conditioning.*

conditioning, respondent See *respondent conditioning.*

conduct disorder A *disruptive behavior disorder* of childhood characterized by repetitive and persistent violation of the rights of others or of age-appropriate social norms or rules. *Symptoms* may include bullying others, truancy or work absences, staying out at night despite parental prohibition before the age of 13, using alcohol or other substances before the age of 13, breaking into another's house or car, firesetting with the intent of causing serious damage, physical cruelty to people or animals, stealing, or use more than once of a weapon that could cause harm to others (e.g., brick, broken bottle, or gun).

confabulation See List of Neurologic Deficits.

confidentiality The ethical principle that a physician may not reveal any information disclosed in the course of medical attendance. See also *privilege* in List of Legal Terms.

conflict A mental struggle that arises from the simultaneous operation of opposing *impulses, drives,* and external (environmental) or internal demands. Termed *intrapsychic* when the conflict is between forces within the personality, and extrapsychic when it is between the self and the environment.

confrontation A communication that deliberately pressures or invites another to self-examine some aspect of behavior in which there is a discrepancy between self-reported and observed behavior.

confusion Disturbed orientation in respect to time, place, or person. See *delirium; dementia; mental status; organic mental disorder.*

congenital Literally, present at birth. It may include conditions that arise during fetal development or with the birth process as well as hereditary or genetically determined conditions. It does not refer to conditions that appear after birth.

conjoint therapy A form of *marital therapy* in which a therapist sees the partners together in joint sessions.

conscience The morally self-critical part of one's standards of behavior, performance, and value judgments. Commonly equated with the *superego*.

conscious The content of mind or mental functioning of which one is aware. In neurology, awake, alert. See also *unconscious*.

conservatorship See LIST OF LEGAL TERMS.

constitution A person's intrinsic physical and psychological endowment; sometimes used more narrowly to indicate physical inheritance or intellectual potential.

constitutional types Constellations of morphological, physiological, and psychological traits as earlier proposed by various scholars. Galen: sanguine, melancholic, choleric, and phlegmatic types; Kretschmer: pyknic (stocky), asthenic (slender), athletic, and dysplastic (disproportioned) types; Sheldon: ectomorphic (thin), mesomorphic (muscular), and endomorphic (fat) types, based on the relative preponderance of outer, middle, or inner layers of embryonic cellular tissue.

constricted affect See *affect*.

consultation-liaison psychiatry An area of special interest in general *psychiatry* that addresses the psychiatric and psychosocial aspects of all medical care, particularly in a general hospital setting. The liaison *psychiatrist* works closely with medical-surgical physicians and nonphysician staff to enhance the diagnosis, treatment, and management of patients with primary medical/surgical illness and concurrent psychiatric disorders or *symptoms*. Consultation may be to any part of the health care system that affects the patient and the family. It may occasionally lead to a recommendation for more specific aftercare referral, but more typically consists of short-term intervention by a "liaison team" with a biopsychosocial approach to illness.

contingency reinforcement In operant or instrumental conditioning, ensuring that desired behavior is followed by positive consequences and that undesired behavior is not rewarded.

continuing medical education (CME) Postgraduate educational activities aimed at maintaining, updating, and extending professional knowledge and skills. Many professional organizations and state licensing boards require participation in CME activities.

contract Explicit commitment between patient and therapist to a well-defined course of action to achieve the treatment goal.

control group See LIST OF RESEARCH TERMS.

conversion A *defense mechanism,* operating unconsciously (see *unconscious*), by which *intrapsychic conflicts* that would otherwise give rise to *anxiety* are instead given symbolic external expression. The repressed ideas or impulses, and the psychological defenses against them, are converted into a variety of somatic *symptoms.* These may include such symptoms as paralysis, pain, or loss of sensory function.

conversion disorder One of the *somatoform disorders* (but in some classifications called a *dissociative disorder*), characterized by a *symptom* suggestive of a neurologic disorder that affects sensation or voluntary motor function. The symptom is not consciously or intentionally produced, it cannot be explained fully by any known *general medical condition,* and it is severe enough to impair functioning or require medical attention. Commonly seen symptoms are blindness, double vision, deafness, impaired coordination, paralysis, and seizures.

convulsive disorders Primarily the centrencephalic seizures, grand mal and petit mal, and the focal seizures of Jacksonian and psychomotor *epilepsy.* These brain disorders, with their characteristic electroencephalographic patterns (see *electroencephalo-*

gram), are to be differentiated from a variety of other pathophysiological conditions in which a convulsive seizure may occur. The latter may follow withdrawal from alcohol, *barbiturates,* and a wide variety of other drugs; they may also occur in cerebral vascular disease, brain tumor, brain abscess, *hypoglycemia,* hyponatremia, and many other metabolic and intracranial disorders.

coordination disorder, developmental A *motor skills disorder* consisting of a level of performance in daily activities requiring motor coordination that is significantly lower than expected, given the subject's age, intelligence, and age-appropriate education. Manifestations include delayed motor milestones (crawling, walking, etc.), clumsiness, and poor handwriting. The term is applied only to presentations that are not due to a general medical condition such as cerebral palsy or muscular dystrophy.

coping mechanisms Ways of adjusting to environmental stress without altering one's goals or purposes; includes both *conscious* and *unconscious* mechanisms.

coprophagia Eating of filth or feces.

coprophilia One of the *paraphilias,* characterized by marked distress over, or acting on, sexual urges involving feces.

core conflictual relationship theme In psychoanalytic therapy (see *psychoanalysis*), any reference by the patient to earlier failures in interpersonal transactions. The patient typically expresses thoughts and feelings about earlier experiences (and especially about parent and child transactions) in a variety of ways, often indirect and veiled. It is the therapist's task to grasp the meaning of the patient's subjective experiences and to understand that the patient's wishes during earlier periods reflected phase-appropriate self-developmental needs and were not simply pleasures to be denied. Such understanding on the part of the therapist will be seen as a validation of the patient's subjective experiences, often earlier denied because of *empathic failures* by the parents.

correlation See LIST OF RESEARCH TERMS.

Cotard's syndrome A nihilistic *delusion* in which one believes that one's body, or parts of it, is disintegrating, or that one is bereft of all resources, or one's family has been exterminated, and so forth. It has been reported in *depressive disorders, schizophrenia,* and lesions of the nondominant lobe. Named after the French *neurologist* Jules Cotard (1840–1887).

counseling A form of supportive *psychotherapy* in which one person, the advisor or counselor, offers guidance or advice to another based on their joint discussion of the other's particular or general personal problems. The method is commonly used by *psychiatrists, psychologists,* social workers, and the clergy.

counterphobia Deliberately seeking out and exposing onself to, rather than avoiding, the object or situation that is consciously or unconsciously feared.

countertransference The therapist's emotional reactions to the patient that are based on the therapist's *unconscious* needs and conflicts, as distinguished from his or her *conscious* responses to the patient's behavior. Countertransference may interfere with the therapist's ability to understand the patient and may adversely affect the therapeutic technique. Currently, there is emphasis on the positive aspects of countertransference and its use as a guide to a more empathic understanding of the patient.

couples therapy See *marital therapy.*

crack Freebase or alkaloidal *cocaine* that is named for the cracking sound it makes when heated. Also known as "rock" for its crystallized appearance. It is ingested by inhalation of vapors produced by heating the "rock." See also TABLE OF COMMONLY ABUSED DRUGS.

cretinism A type of *mental retardation* and bodily malformation caused by severe, uncorrected thyroid deficiency in infancy and early childhood.

cri du chat A type of *mental retardation*. The name is derived from a catlike cry emitted by children with this disorder, which is caused by partial deletion of chromosome 5.

crisis A state of sudden psychological disequilibrium; turning point in a person's life.

crisis intervention A form of *brief psychotherapy* that emphasizes identification of the specific event precipitating the emotional trauma and uses methods to neutralize that trauma. Often used in hospital emergency rooms.

cross-cultural psychiatry The comparative study of *mental illness* and *mental health* among different societies, nations, and cultures. Often used synonymously with transcultural psychiatry.

cross-dependence A drug's ability to suppress physical manifestations of substance dependence produced by another drug and to maintain the physically dependent state. It provides the rationale for the treatment of dependence on one substance, such as alcohol, by short-term substitution of a less dangerous and more controllable substance that is cross-dependent with alcohol (e.g., diazepam).

cross-dressing See *transvestism*.

cross-tolerance Tolerance to a drug to which the subject has not been exposed, by reason of tolerance developed to another substance over a period of long-term administration. A person who has developed tolerance to alcohol will not respond to the usual dose of volative anesthetic because tolerance to alcohol has also induced tolerance to the anesthetic.

cult A system of beliefs and rituals based on dogma or religious teachings that are usually contrary to the ones established within or accepted by the community.

cultural anthropology The study of human society with emphasis on how values, customs, beliefs, language, and other patterns of behavior are transmitted by learning from past generations. See *ethnology; social anthropology*.

cultural psychiatry A branch of *social psychiatry* concerned with mentally ill persons in relation to their cultural environment. *Symptoms* of behavior regarded as psychopathological in one society may be regarded as acceptable and normal in another.

culture shock Feelings of isolation, rejection, and alienation experienced by an individual or group when transplanted from a familiar to an unfamiliar culture (e.g., from one country to another).

culture-specific syndromes Forms of disturbed behavior specific to certain cultural systems that do not conform to western nosologic entities (see *nosology*). Some commonly cited syndromes are the following:

Syndrome	Culture	Symptoms
amok	Malay	Acute indiscriminate homicidal mania
koro	China, Southeast Asia	Fear of retraction of penis into abdomen with the belief that this will lead to death
latah	Southeast Asia	Startle-induced disorganization, hypersuggestibility, automatic obedience, and *echopraxia*
piblokto	Eskimo	Attacks of screaming, crying, and running naked through the snow
windigo	Canadian	*Delusions* of being possessed by a cannabalistic monster (*windigo*), attacks of agitated *depression,* oral sadistic fears and impulses

See *trance disorder, dissociative*.

CVA Cerebrovascular accident. See *stroke*.

cyclothymic disorder In DSM-IV, one of the *bipolar disorders* characterized by numerous hypomanic episodes and frequent periods of depressed mood or loss of interest or pleasure. These episodes do not meet the criteria for a full manic episode or major depressive disorder. See *depressive disorders*.

D

Da Costa's syndrome Neurocirculatory asthenia; "soldier's heart"; a functional disorder of the circulatory system that is usually a part of an *anxiety* state or secondary to *hyperventilation*.

day hospital See *partial hospitalization*.

day residue Any element of a dream that is clearly derived from some event of the previous day.

death instinct (Thanatos) In Freudian theory, the *unconscious* drive toward dissolution and death. Coexists with and is in opposition to the life *instinct* (Eros).

decompensation The deterioration of existing defenses (see *defense mechanism*), leading to an exacerbation of pathological behavior.

defense mechanism *Unconscious* intrapsychic processes serving to provide relief from emotional *conflict* and *anxiety*. *Conscious* efforts are frequently made for the same reasons, but true defense mechanisms are unconscious. Some of the common defense mechanisms defined in this glossary are *compensation, conversion, denial, displacement, dissociation, idealization, identification, incorporation, introjection, projection, rationalization, reaction formation, re-*

54

gression, sublimation, substitution, symbolization, and *undoing.*

deficit Insufficient quantity or inadequate supply. In *neurology* it refers to inability to perform (e.g., a motor action) because of some interference along the chain of neurophysiological and neurochemical events that lies between stimulus and response.

deficit schizophrenia See *schizophrenia.*

deinstitutionalization Change in locus of mental health care from traditional, institutional settings to community-based services. Sometimes called trans-institutionalization because it often merely shifts the patients from one institution (the hospital) to another (such as a prison).

déjà vu A paramnesia consisting of the sensation or illusion that one is seeing what one has seen before.

delayed sleep phase See *circadian rhythm sleep disorder.*

delirium A *cognitive disorder* characterized by impairment in consciousness, attention, and changes in cognition (e.g., memory deficit, disorientation, language or perceptual disturbance). The following types of delirium are recognized by DSM-IV: delirium due to a general medical condition, substance-induced delirium (in intoxication and withdrawal states), delirium due to multiple etiologies, and delirium of unknown etiology or not otherwise specified.

delirium tremens Alcohol withdrawal *delirium;* alcohol delirium with onset during withdrawal. See *withdrawal symptoms, alcohol.*

delusion A false belief based on an incorrect inference about external reality and firmly sustained despite clear evidence to the contrary. The belief is not part of a cultural tradition such as an article of religious faith. Among the more frequently reported delusions are the following:

delusion of control The belief that one's feelings, impulses, thoughts, or actions are not one's own but have been imposed by some external force.

delusion of poverty The conviction that one is, or will be, bereft of all material possessions.

delusion of reference The conviction that events, objects, or other people in the immediate environment have a particular and unusual significance (usually negative).

delusional jealousy The false belief that one's sexual partner is unfaithful; also called the Othello delusion.

grandiose delusion An exaggerated belief of one's importance, power, knowledge, or identity.

nihilistic delusion A conviction of nonexistence of the self, part of the self, or others, or of the world. "I no longer have a brain" is an example.

persecutory delusion The conviction that one (or a group or institution close to one) is being harassed, attacked, persecuted, or conspired against.

somatic delusion A false belief involving the functioning of one's body, such as the conviction of a postmenopausal woman that she is pregnant, or a person's conviction that his nose is misshapen and ugly when there is nothing wrong with it.

systematized delusion A single false belief with multiple elaborations or a group of false beliefs that the person relates to a single event or theme. This event is believed to have caused every problem in life that the person experiences.

delusional depression Severe *depressive disorder* characterized by psychotic thinking (e.g., *delusions* or *hallucinations*) as well as neurovegetative symptoms. Listed in DSM-IV as major depression with psychotic features.

delusional disorder A paranoid disorder; although in practice often difficult to differentiate from *paranoid* *schizophrenia,* the delusions in this disorder are characteristically systematized and not bizarre, other characteristics of the active phase of schizophrenia are absent or only fleetingly present, personality functioning remains relatively intact outside the area of the delusional theme, and overall impairment remains less than in schizophrenia.

Subtypes are recognized on the basis of the predominant delusional theme: erotomanic (i.e., the delusion that another person, usually of higher status, is in love with the person); grandiose (i.e., delusions of inflated worth, power, knowledge, or identity); jealous (i.e., the delusion that one's sexual partner is unfaithful); persecutory (i.e., the delusion that one, or someone to whom one is close, is being treated malevolently); somatic (i.e., the delusion that one has some physical defect or nonpsychiatric medical condition); and mixed.

dementia   A *cognitive disorder* characterized by defects in *memory, aphasia, apraxia, agnosia,* and executive functioning.

Various forms of dementia are recognized in DSM-IV: 1) dementia due to a general medical condition, including dementia of the *Alzheimer* type; *dementia, vascular; HIV dementia;* and dementia due to *Pick's disease, Creutzfeldt-Jakob disease, Huntington's disease,* and *Parkinson's disease;* 2) substance-induced persisting dementia (seen with alcohol, inhalants, and sedatives/hypnotics/ anxiolytics); 3) dementia due to multiple etiologies; 4) dementia of unknown etiology; and 5) dementia not otherwise specified.

dementia, senile   See *senile dementia.*

dementia, vascular   Also known as multi-infarct dementia, *cerebral arteriosclerosis. Dementia* with focal neurologic signs and *symptoms.* Typically, the course is one of a period of clinical stability punctuated by sudden significant cognitive and functional losses (stepwise deterioration).

dementia praecox Obsolete descriptive term for *schizophrenia.* Introduced as "démence précoce" by Morel (1857) and later popularized by *Kraepelin.*

demography The study of a population and those variables bringing about change in that population. See also *epidemiology.*

dendrite A branch of the nerve cell that receives nerve impulses from the *axon* of a neighboring nerve; a tree-like extension of the neuron cell body. It receives information, along with the cell body, from other neurons.

denial A *defense mechanism,* operating unconsciously, used to resolve emotional *conflict* and allay *anxiety* by disavowing thoughts, feelings, wishes, needs, or external reality factors that are consciously intolerable.

deoxyribonucleic acid (DNA) Chemical substance found in *chromosomes* within cell nuclei; its molecular structure contains the organism's genetic information.

dependence Reliance on someone or something else for support. In *psychiatry,* used to refer to needs for protection, security, food, and so forth, as in the child's dependence on a caregiver (see *dependent personality disorder*). It also applies to the substance-abusing person's need to continue use of the psychoactive substance; see *dependence, substance.*

dependence, substance *Chemical dependence;* sometimes defined in terms of physiological dependence as evidenced by *tolerance* or *withdrawal;* at other times defined in terms of impairment in social and occupational functioning resulting from the pathological and repeated use of a substance. In the latter, tolerance and withdrawal symptoms may be present but are not essential.

The behaviors and effects associated with substance dependence include taking of the substance to relieve or avoid withdrawal symptoms; taking of larger amounts or using over a longer period than intended; unsuccessful efforts to cut down or control intake; interference with meeting major role obligations at work, school, or home; recurrent use in situations when it poses a physical hazard (e.g., driving, operating machinery); or substance use taking precedence over important social, occupational, or recreational activities.

dependency needs Vital needs for mothering, love, affection, shelter, protection, security, food, and warmth. May be a manifestation of *regression* when they reappear openly in adults.

dependent personality disorder Disorder characterized by a lack of self-confidence, a tendency to have others assume responsibility for one's life, and subordination of one's needs and wishes to the person(s) on whom one is dependent. See *personality disorder*.

depersonalization Feelings of unreality or strangeness concerning either the environment, the self, or both. This is characteristic of *depersonalization disorder* and may also occur in *schizotypal personality disorder, schizophrenia,* and in those persons experiencing overwhelming *anxiety,* stress, or fatigue.

depersonalization disorder One of the *dissociative disorders,* characterized by persistent or recurrent feelings of being detached from one's body or mental processes. The affected person often complains of being an automaton or an outside observer of his or her self.

depression When used to describe a *mood,* depression refers to feelings of sadness, despair, and discouragement. As such, depression may be a normal feeling state. The overt manifestations are highly variable and may be *culture specific.* Depression may be a *symptom* seen in a variety of mental or physical disorders, a *syndrome* of associated symptoms secondary to an underlying disorder, or a specific *mental disorder*. Slowed thinking, decreased pleasure, decreased purposeful physical activity, *guilt* and hopelessness, and disorders of eating and sleeping may be seen in the depressive syndrome. DSM-IV classifies depression by severity, recurrence, and association with *hypomania* or *mania*. Other categorizations divide depression into reactive and endogenous depressions on the basis of precipitants or symptom clusters. Depression in children may be indicated by refusal to go to school, *anxiety,* excessive reaction to separation from parental figures, antisocial behavior, and somatic complaints.

depression with psychotic features Major depressive episode with *delusions* or *hallucinations* whose content may be consistent with the depressive themes of inadequacy, *guilt,* disease, or death. Sometimes such features as persecutory *delusions,* thought insertion, thought broadcasting, and *delusions of control* may be present.

depressive disorders In DSM-IV, a group of *mood disorders* that includes major depressive disorder (single episode or recurrent); *dysthymic disorder;* and depressive disorder not otherwise specified (NOS).

major depressive disorder (in other classificatory systems called major depression; manic-depressive disorder, depressed) occurs in a person who has never had an episode of *mania* and is characterized by significant lowering of the mood tone and loss of interest or pleasure in daily activities, plus a range of other *symptoms* that may include significant weight or appetite changes, *insomnia* or *hypersomnia, psychomotor agitation* or retardation, fatigue or loss of energy, feelings of worthlessness or excessive and inappropriate *guilt,* diminished ability to think or concentrate, indecisiveness, and recurrent thoughts of death or *suicide.* Some patients have only a single episode, whereas others have recurrent episodes of depression.

depressive disorder not otherwise specified (NOS) includes *premenstrual dysphoric disorder* and postpsychotic depression of *schizophrenia.*

depressive personality disorder Used by some investigators to refer to persistent, enduring characteristic mood tone that is gloomy, cheerless, unhappy, or dejected. The person's self concepts include persistent beliefs of inadequacy, worthlessness, and low self-esteem. Attitudes toward others are negative, critical, and judgmental. The person is brooding, worrisome, pessimistic, and prone to feelings of guilt. As described, such a personality disorder overlaps considerably with the concept of *dysthymic disorder.*

depressive position A term applied by Melanie *Klein* and her followers to the stage of development that peaks about the sixth month of life. The infant begins to fear destroying and losing the beloved object and wants to appease it and preserve it.

depressive-anxiety disorder, mixed See *mixed anxiety-depressive disorder.*

deprivation, emotional Lack of adequate and appropriate interpersonal and/or environmental experience, usually in the early developmental years.

deprivation, sensory See *sensory deprivation.*

depth psychology An inexact term referring to the *psychology* of *unconscious* mental processes. Also a system of psychology in which the study of such processes plays a major role, as in *psychoanalysis.*

derealization A feeling of estrangement or detachment from one's environment. May be accompanied by *depersonalization.*

dereflection See *existential psychotherapy.*

dereistic Mental activity that is not in accordance with reality, logic, or experience. See also *autism.*

descriptive psychiatry A system of *psychiatry* based on the study of readily observable external factors. Often used to refer to the systematized descriptions of mental illness formulated by *Kraepelin*. Contrast with *dynamic psychiatry*.

desensitization See *systematic desensitization*.

designer drugs Addictive drugs that are synthesized or manufactured to give the same subjective effects as well-known illicit drugs. Because the process is a covert operation, there is difficulty in tracing the manufacturer to check the drugs for adverse effects. Common examples are "ecstacy" and "eve," both of which are similar to *amphetamines*.

desire disorder, sexual See *sexual desire disorders*.

desynchronized sleep rhythm See *circadian rhythm sleep disorder*.

detachment A behavior pattern characterized by general aloofness in interpersonal contact; may include *intellectualization, denial,* and superficiality.

determinism The theory that one's emotional life does not result from chance alone but rather from specific causes or forces, known or unknown.

detoxification The process of providing medical care during the removal of dependence-producing substances from the body so that *withdrawal symptoms* are minimized and physiological function is safely restored. Treatment includes medication, rest, diet, fluids, and nursing care.

devaluation In *psychiatry,* a mental mechanism in which one attributes exaggeratedly negative qualities to oneself or others.

developmental lines The different stages through which an organism passes during its life span, often described separately for different organ systems or functions. Each stage usually shows characteristic features and presents its own challenges that must be met if development is to proceed normally.

deviation, sexual   See *paraphilias.*

diagnosis   The process of determining, through examination and analysis, the nature of a patient's illness.

***Diagnostic and Statistical Manual of Mental Disorders* (DSM)**   The *American Psychiatric Association*'s official classification of mental disorders.

   DSM-I   The first edition, published in 1952.

   DSM-II   The second edition, published in 1968.

   DSM-III   The third edition, published in 1980.

   DSM-III-R   The revised DSM-III, published in 1987.

   DSM-IV   The fourth edition, published in 1994.

diagnostic related groups (DRG)   Medical-based classification, representing 23 major diagnostic categories, that aggregates patients into case types based on diagnosis. A diagnosis related group is a subset of a major diagnostic category.

differential diagnosis   The consideration of which of two or more diseases with similar *symptoms* the patient suffers from.

differentiation   The degree to which an individual identifies the self as separate or distinct from others. See *separation-individuation.*

diplopia   Double vision due to paralysis of the ocular muscles; seen in inhalant intoxication and other conditions affecting the oculomotor nerve.

disability (psychiatric)   Deprivation of intellectual or emotional capacity or fitness. As defined by the federal government, "Inability to engage in any substantial gainful activity by reason of any medically determinable physical or mental impairment which can be expected to last or has lasted for a continuous period of not less than 12 full months."

disconnection syndrome   Term coined by Norman Geschwind (1926–1984) to describe the interruption of information transferred from one brain region to another.

discordance   See LIST OF RESEARCH TERMS.

disinhibition Freedom to act according to one's inner drives or feelings, with less regard for restraints imposed by cultural norms or one's *superego;* removal of an inhibitory, constraining, or limiting influence, as in the escape from higher cortical control in neurologic injury, or in uncontrolled firing of impulses, as when a drug interferes with the usual limiting or inhibiting action of *GABA* within the *central nervous system.*

disintegration anxiety See *fragmentation.*

disintegrative disorder A developmental disorder of childhood characterized by normal development for at least the first 2 years of life followed by loss of previously acquired skills in two or more of the following: expressive or receptive language, social skills or adaptive behavior, bowel or bladder control, play, and motor skills. In addition, there is gross impairment in social interaction and communication, and restricted patterns of behavior, interest, and activities, all similar to manifestations described in *autistic disorder.*

disorientation Loss of awareness of the position of the self in relation to space, time, or other persons; confusion. See also *delirium; dementia.*

displacement A *defense mechanism,* operating unconsciously (see *unconscious*), in which emotions, ideas, or wishes are transferred from their original object to a more acceptable substitute; often used to allay *anxiety.*

disruptive behavior and attention-deficit disorders In DSM-IV, this group includes *attention-deficit/hyperactivity disorder, conduct disorder,* and *oppositional defiant disorder.*

disruptive behavior disorder A disturbance of conduct severe enough to produce significant impairment in social, occupational, or academic functioning because of *symptoms* that range from oppositional defiant to moderate and severe conduct disturbances.

oppositional defiant symptoms may include losing temper; arguing with adults and actively refusing their requests; deliberately annoying others; blaming others for one's mistakes; being easily annoyed, resentful, or spiteful; and physically fighting with other members of the household.

conduct disturbance (moderate) symptoms may include truancy or work absences, alcohol or other substance use before the age of 13, stealing with confrontation, destruction of others' property, firesetting with intent of causing serious damage, initiating fights outside of home, and being physically cruel to animals.

conduct disturbance (severe) symptoms may include running away from home overnight at least twice, breaking into another's property, being physically cruel to people, stealing with confrontation, repeatedly using a dangerous weapon, and forcing someone into sexual activity.

dissociation The splitting off of clusters of mental contents from *conscious* awareness, a mechanism central to hysterical conversion and *dissociative disorders;* the separation of an idea from its emotional significance and affect as seen in the inappropriate *affect* of schizophrenic patients.

dissociative disorder, brief reactive See *stress disorder, acute.*

dissociative disorders In DSM-IV, this category includes dissociative *amnesia,* dissociative *fugue,* dissociative identity disorder (*multiple personality disorder*), and *depersonalization disorder.* Included within dissociative disorders not otherwise specified are dissociative trance disorder and *Ganser's syndrome.*

distractibility Inability to maintain attention; shifting from one area or topic to another with minimal provocation. Distractibility may be a manifestation of organic impairment or it may be a part of a functional disorder such as an *anxiety disorder, mania,* or *schizophrenia.*

distributive analysis and synthesis The therapy used by the psychobiological school of psychiatry developed by *Meyer;* entails extensive guided and directed investigation and analysis of the patient's entire past experience, stressing assets and liabilities to make possible a constructive synthesis. See *psychobiology.*

Dix, Dorothea Lynde (1802–1887) Foremost 19th-century American crusader for the improvement of institutional care of the mentally ill.

dizygotic twins Twins who develop from two separately fertilized ova. Also called fraternal twins.

DNA See *deoxyribonucleic acid.*

dominance A predisposition to play a prominent or controlling role when interacting with others. In *neurology,* the (normal) tendency of one-half of the brain to be more important than the other in mediating various functions (cerebral dominance). In genetics, the ability of one *gene* (dominant gene) to express itself in the *phenotype* of an individual when paired with another (recessive) gene that would have expressed itself in a different way.

dopamine (3,4-dihydroxyphenethylamine) A synaptic *neurotransmitter* found in the brain, specifically associated with some forms of *psychosis* and movement disorders. See also *biogenic amines.*

dopamine hypothesis A theory that attempts to explain the pathogenesis of *schizophrenia* and other psychotic states as due to excesses in *dopamine* activity in various areas of the brain. This theory is, in part, based on biological observations that the antipsychotic properties of specific drugs may be related to their ability to block the action of dopamine, and the opposite effects of stimulants that increase the action of dopamine.

double bind   Interaction in which one person demands a response to a message containing mutually contradictory signals, while the other person is unable either to comment on the incongruity or to escape from the situation.

double-blind   See LIST OF RESEARCH TERMS.

double personality   See *multiple personality disorder.*

Down syndrome   Also known as trisomy 21, a common form of *mental retardation* caused by a chromosomal abnormality; formerly called mongolism. Two types are recognized, based on the nature of the chromosomal aberration: the translocation type and the nondisjunction type. Physical findings include widely spaced eyes with slanting openings, small head with flattened occiput, lax joints, flabby hands, small ears, and *congenital* anomalies of the heart. See also *chromosome 21.*

dream anxiety disorder   *Nightmare disorder.* See *parasomnias.*

DRG based payments   See *diagnostic related groups.*

drive   Basic urge, instinct, motivation; a term used to avoid confusion with the more purely biological concept of *instinct.*

drug abuse   See *drug dependence.*

drug dependence   Habituation to, abuse of, and/or *addiction* to a chemical substance. Largely because of psychological craving, the life of the drug-dependent person revolves around the need for the specific effect of one or more chemical agents on *mood* or state of consciousness. The term thus includes not only the addiction (which emphasizes the physiological dependence) but also drug abuse (in which the pathological craving for drugs seems unrelated to physical dependence). Examples include alcohol, *opiates,* synthetic analgesics with morphine-like effects, *barbiturates,* other hypnotics, sedatives, some antianxiety agents, *cocaine,* psychostimulants, marijuana, and *psychoto-mimetic* drugs.

drug holiday   Discontinuance of a therapeutic drug for a limited period of time. Sometimes used as a way of evaluating baseline behavior or as a means of controlling or reducing the dosage of psychoactive drugs and side effects.

drug interaction   The effects of two or more drugs taken simultaneously, producing an alteration in the usual effects of either drug taken alone. The interacting drugs may have a potentiating or additive effect and serious side effects may result. An example of drug interaction is alcohol and *sedative* drugs taken together, leading to intensification of *central nervous system* depression.

drug levels   See *blood levels.*

drug tolerance   See *tolerance.*

drug-induced parkinsonism (pseudoparkinsonism)   A *syndrome* resembling Parkinson's disease, resulting from the *dopamine*-blocking action of antipsychotic drugs. Pill-rolling movements are less common in this syndrome than in the naturally occurring disorder.

DSM   See *Diagnostic and Statistical Manual of Mental Disorders.*

dual addiction   Coexisting substance abuse and mental illness.

dual diagnosis   The co-occurrence within one's lifetime of a psychiatric disorder and a *substance use disorder. Comorbidity* is the preferred term.

dummy   British term for *placebo.*

dura mater   The outermost of the meninges that covers the brain and spinal cord. The subdural space lies below it and separates it from the arachnoid membrane.

Durham rule   See under *insanity defense* in List of Legal Terms.

dyad A two-person relationship, such as the therapeutic relationship between doctor and patient in individual *psychotherapy*.

dynamic psychiatry The study of *psychiatry* from the point of view of motivation, emphasizing both psychological meaning and biological instincts as forces relevant to understanding human behavior in health, as well as illness. Contrast with *descriptive psychiatry*.

dynamics See *psychodynamics*.

dys- See LIST OF NEUROLOGIC DEFICITS.

dysarthria Difficulty in speech production due to lack of coordination of the speech apparatus. See LIST OF NEUROLOGIC DEFICITS.

dyscalculia See *learning disability*.

dysgraphia See *learning disability*.

dyskinesia Any disturbance of movement. It may also be induced by medication.

dyskinesia, tardive See *tardive dyskinesia*.

dyslexia Inability or difficulty in reading, including word-blindness and a tendency to reverse letters and words in reading and writing. See *learning disability*. See also *alexia* in LIST OF NEUROLOGIC DEFICITS.

dysmnesia General intellectual impairment secondary to defects of memory and orientation. See also *organic mental disorder*.

dysmnesic syndrome See *dysmnesia*.

dyspareunia One of the *sexual pain disorders*.

dysphagia Difficult or painful swallowing.

dysphonia Disorder of speech due to dysfunction of vocal cords.

dysphoria Unpleasant *mood*.

dysphoric disorder, late luteal phase See *premenstrual dysphoric disorder*.

dyssocial behavior The behavior of persons who are not classifiable as antisocial personalities but who are predatory and follow criminal pursuits. Formerly called sociopathic personalities. See also *personality disorder.*

dyssomnias A major subgroup of *sleep disorders* (*parasomnias* are the other major subgroup) in which the predominant disturbance is in the amount, quality, or timing of sleep. In DSM-IV, this group includes primary *insomnia,* primary *hypersomnia, narcolepsy, breathing-related sleep disorder,* and *circadian rhythm sleep disorder.* Nocturnal myoclonus is classified as a sleep disorder not otherwise specified; it consists of repeated jerking of the limbs, particularly the legs, associated with brief periods of arousal.

dysthymic disorder One of the *depressive disorders,* characterized by a chronic course (i.e., seldom without *symptoms*) with lowered *mood* tone and a range of other symptoms that may include feelings of inadequacy, loss of self-esteem, or self-deprecation; feelings of hopelessness or despair; feelings of *guilt,* brooding about past events, or self-pity; low energy and chronic tiredness; being less active or talkative than usual; poor concentration and indecisiveness; and inability to enjoy pleasurable activities.

dystonia, acute, neuroleptic-induced Abnormal positioning or spasm of the muscles of the head, neck, limbs, or trunk; the dystonia develops within a few days of starting or raising the dose of a neuroleptic medication, because of dysfunction of the *extrapyramidal system.*

E

EAP See *employee assistance program.*

eating disorder Marked disturbance in eating behavior. In DSM-IV, this category includes *anorexia* *nervosa, bulimia nervosa,* and eating disorder not otherwise specified.

echolalia Parrot-like repetition of overheard words or fragments of speech. It may be part of a developmental disorder, a neurologic disorder, or *schizophrenia.* Echolalia tends to be repetitive and persistent and is often uttered with a mocking, mumbling, or staccato intonation. See also LIST OF NEUROLOGIC DEFICITS.

echopraxia Imitative repetition of the movements, gestures, or posture of another. It may be part of a neurologic disorder or of *schizophrenia.*

ecology The study of the mutual relationship between people and their environment.

economic viewpoint One of three metapsychological positions explicitly formulated by *Freud* concerned with the distribution, transformations, and expenditure of psychic energy.

ecopsychiatry Scientific concept describing the basic and applied relationship between living things and their environment. These are assumed, by their presence or absence, to affect mental health.

ECT See *electroconvulsive therapy.*

ectomorphic See *constitutional types.*

educable Capable of achieving a fourth- or fifth-grade academic level; mildly mentally retarded (IQ of 52 to 67). See *mental retardation.*

EEG See *electroencephalogram.*

ego In psychoanalytic theory (see *psychoanalysis*), one of the three major divisions in the model of the psychic apparatus, the others being the *id* and the *superego.* The ego represents the sum of certain mental mechanisms, such as perception and memory, and specific *defense mechanisms.* It serves to mediate between the demands of primitive instinctual drives (the id), of internalized parental and social prohibitions (the superego), and of reality. The compromises between these forces achieved by the ego tend to resolve intrapsychic *conflict* and serve an adaptive and executive function. Psychiatric usage of the term should not be confused with common usage, which connotes self-love or selfishness.

ego analysis Intensive psychoanalytic study and analysis of the ways in which the *ego* resolves or attempts to deal with intrapsychic *conflicts,* especially in relation to the development of mental mechanisms and the maturation of capacity for rational thought and action. Modern *psychoanalysis* gives more emphasis to considerations of the defensive operations of the ego than did earlier techniques, which emphasized *instinctual* forces to a greater degree.

ego boundaries Hypothesized lines of demarcation between the ego and 1) the external world (external ego boundary) and 2) the internal world, including the repressed *unconscious,* the *id,* and much of the *superego* (internal ego boundary).

ego ideal The part of the personality that comprises the aims and goals for the self; usually refers to the *conscious* or *unconscious* emulation of significant figures with whom one has identified. The ego ideal emphasizes what one should be or do in contrast to what one should not be or not do.

ego psychology The study and elucidation of those slowly changing functions known as psychic structures that usually shape, channel, and organize mental activity into meaningful and tolerable patterns of experience. The usual structures referred to in this sense are memory, speech, locomotion, cognition, drive, restraint, discharge, and the capacity to make judgments and decisions. See *Freud, Sigmund.*

ego strength The ability of the ego to execute its functions, to mediate between the external world, the *id,* and the *superego* effectively and efficiently, so that energy is left over for creativity and other integrative activities. Among specific functions that may be assessed in determining ego strength are judgment, *reality testing,* regulation of drives, defensive functions, thought processes, and object relations.

ego-alien See *ego-dystonic.*

egocentric Self-centered.

ego-dystonic Referring to aspects of a person's behavior, thoughts, and attitudes that are viewed by the self as repugnant or inconsistent with the total *personality.* Contrast to *ego-syntonic.*

egomania See under *-mania.*

ego-syntonic Referring to aspects of a person's behavior, thoughts, and attitudes that are viewed by the self as acceptable and consistent with the total *personality.* Contrast to *ego-dystonic.*

eidetic image Unusually vivid and apparently exact mental image; may be a memory, *fantasy,* or dream.

ejaculatio retardata See *orgasm disorders.*

ejaculatory incompetence (impotence) Inability to reach orgasm and ejaculate despite adequacy of erection. See *orgasm disorders.*

elaboration An *unconscious* process consisting of expansion and embellishment of detail, especially with reference to a symbol or representation in a dream.

elective mutism See *mutism, selective.*

Electra complex The female *Oedipus complex;* an infrequently used term describing the pathological relationship between a woman and a man based on unresolved developmental *conflicts.*

electroconvulsive therapy (ECT) Use of electric current with anesthetics and muscle relaxants to induce convulsive seizures. Most effective in the treatment of *depression.* Introduced by Cerletti and Bini in 1938. Modifications are electronarcosis, which produces sleeplike states, and electrostimulation, which avoids convulsions.

electroencephalogram (EEG) A graphic (voltage vs. time) depiction of the brain's electrical potentials (brain waves) recorded by scalp electrodes. It is used for diagnosis in neurologic and neuropsychiatric disorders and in neurophysiological research. Sometimes used interchangeably with electrocorticogram and depth record, in which the electrodes are in direct contact with brain tissue.

electromyogram (EMG) An electrophysiological recording of muscle potentials that measures the amount and nature of muscle activity at the site from which the recording is taken.

electroshock treatment (EST) See *electroconvulsive therapy*.

electrostimulation See *electroconvulsive therapy*.

elimination disorders Included in this group are functional *encopresis* and functional *enuresis*.

elopement A patient's unauthorized departure from a psychiatric facility.

emergence See *epigenesis*.

EMG See *electromyogram*.

emotion A state of arousal determined by a set of subjective feelings, often accompanied by physiological changes, that impels one toward action. Examples are fear, anger, love, and hate. See *affect*.

emotional control therapies See *experiential therapy*.

emotional disturbance See *mental disorder*.

emotional illness See *mental disorder*.

emotional release therapies See *experiential therapy*.

empathic failure Lack of responsivity to a child's phase-appropriate needs. In a treatment setting, a therapist's lack of responsivity to the patient. See *holding environment; mirroring*.

empathy Insightful awareness, including the meaning and significance of the feelings, *emotions,* and behavior of another person. Contrast with *sympathy*.

employee assistance program (EAP) Confidential help provided by companies and other employers to their employees for personal problems that might influence their ability to work effectively. Programs started in the early 1900s as employee counseling, switched in the 1960s to helping employees who were having problems with alcohol, and were expanded subsequently to include other personal problems.

encephalitis Either acute or chronic inflammation of the brain caused by viruses, bacteria, spirochetes, fungi, or protozoa. Neurologic signs and *symptoms* and various mental and behavioral changes occur during the illness and may persist. See also *encephalopathy; organic mental disorder.*

encephalopathy An imprecise term referring to any disorder of brain function (metabolic, toxic, neoplastic), but often implying a chronic degenerative process.

encopresis, functional An elimination disorder in a child who is at least 4 years of age, consisting of repeated passage of feces into inappropriate places (clothing, floor, etc.) and not due to a *general medical condition.*

encounter group therapy See *experiential therapy.*

endemic See under *epidemiology.*

endocrine disorders Disturbances of the function of the ductless glands that may be metabolic in origin and may be associated with or aggravated by emotional factors, producing mental and behavioral disturbances in addition to physical signs.

Of particular significance in *psychiatry* is the hypothalamic-pituitary-adrenal (HPA) axis, consisting of a self-regulating circle of neurohormones released from the *hypothalamus* and stimulating the release of hormones from the anterior pituitary. These in turn stimulate hormone secretion in target organs (thyroid, adrenal, and gonads). The HPA axis is involved in the regulation of sexual activity, thirst and hunger behaviors, sleep, learning and memory, and perhaps in antidepressant activity.

endogenous Originating or beginning within the organism.

endogenous depression See *depression.*

endogenous psychoses The various forms of *schizophrenia* and *mood disorders,* and primary degenerative disorders of the *central nervous system* that, so far as it is known, arise within the organism itself. Contrast to *exogenous psychoses.*

endomorphic See *constitutional types.*

endorphin One family of endogenous brain peptides with morphine-like action; the other brain opioids are dynorphin and the *enkephalins.* The endorphins modulate pain perception and possibly mood and response to stress.

engram A memory trace; a neurophysiological process that accounts for persistence of memory.

enkephalin Endogenous opioid peptide found in the brain. See *endorphin.*

entitlement The right or claim to something. In health law, entitlement programs refer to legislatively defined rights to health care, such as Medicare and Medicaid programs.

In psychodynamic *psychiatry,* entitlement usually refers to an unreasonable expectation or unfounded claim. An example is a person with *narcissistic personality disorder* who feels deserving of preferred status and special treatment even though there is no apparent justification for such treatment.

enuresis, functional An elimination disorder in a child who is at least 5 years of age, consisting of repeated voiding of urine into bed or clothing, and not due to any *general medical condition.*

enzyme An organic compound that interacts with a biological substrate to form a new chemical, either (and more commonly) through the process of synthesis or through degradation. For example, the enzyme *monoamine oxidase* degrades *biogenic amines.*

epidemiology In *psychiatry,* the study of the incidence, distribution, prevalence, and control of *mental disorders* in a given population. Common terms in epidemiology are

endemic Native to or restricted to a particular area.

epidemic The outbreak of a disorder that affects significant numbers of persons in a given population at any time.

pandemic Occurring over a very wide area, in many countries, or universally.

See also *incidence, period prevalence,* and *point prevalence* in LIST OF RESEARCH TERMS.

epigenesis Originally from the Greek *epi* (on, upon, on top of) and "genesis" (origin); the theory that the embryo is not preformed in the ovum or the sperm, but that it develops gradually by the successive formation of new parts. The concept has been extended to other areas of medicine, with different shades of meaning. Some of the other meanings are as follows:

1. Any change in an organism that is due to outside influences rather than to genetically determined ones.
2. The occurrence of secondary *symptoms* as a result of disease.
3. Developmental factors, and specifically the gene-environment interactions, that contribute to development.
4. The appearance of new functions that are not predictable on the basis of knowledge of the part-processes that have been combined.
5. The appearance of specific features at each stage of development, such as the different goals and risks that *Erikson* described for the eight stages of human life (trust vs. mistrust, autonomy vs. doubt,

etc.). The life cycle theory adheres to the epigenetic principle in that each stage of development is characterized by crises or challenges that must be satisfactorily resolved if development is to proceed normally.

epigenetics The study of the factors that cause development. See *epigenesis*.

epilepsy A neurologic disorder characterized by periodic motor or sensory seizures or their equivalents, sometimes accompanied by alterations of consciousness. The *electroencephalogram* may show an abnormal brain wave pattern during or between seizures. Idiopathic epilepsy is of no known organic cause; epilepsy is termed symptomatic when it is secondary to organic lesions.

Epilepsy is generally divided into partial or general seizures. In partial seizures, consciousness may not be impaired. In seizures with complex symptoms (*temporal lobe epilepsy, psychomotor* seizures), consciousness usually is impaired. Among the many forms of generalized seizures are absences (formerly called petit mal epilepsy) and tonic-clonic seizures (formerly called grand mal seizures). Status epilepticus refers to prolongation of a grand mal seizure and its failure to end spontaneously.

epileptic equivalent Episodic, sensory, or motor phenomena that a person with epilepsy may experience instead of convulsive seizures.

Jacksonian epilepsy A type of grand mal epilepsy that typically begins with convulsive seizures (clonic) and movements of the thumb and forefinger, or the angle of the mouth, or the big toe, and spreads to include the rest of the limb and finally the other side of the body. At this point, consciousness is usually lost. Named after neurologist J. Hughlings Jackson (1835–1911).

major epilepsy (grand mal) Gross convulsive seizures with loss of consciousness and vegetative control.

minor epilepsy (petit mal) Nonconvulsive epileptic seizures or equivalents; may be limited only to momentary lapses of consciousness.

temporal lobe epilepsy Also called complex partial seizures. Usually originating in the temporal lobes, it involves recurrent periodic disturbances of behavior, during which the patient carries out movements that are often repetitive and highly organized but semiautomatic in character. See *interictal behavior syndrome.*

epinephrine One of the *catecholamines* secreted by the adrenal gland and by fibers of the *sympathetic nervous system.* It is responsible for many of the physical manifestations of *fear* and *anxiety.* Also known as adrenalin.

epistemology The theory of knowledge; the study of the method and grounds of knowledge.

erectile disorder One of the *sexual arousal disorders.*

Erikson, Erik H. (1902–) German-born lay *psychoanalyst* and child psychoanalyst noted for his work on *psychosocial development;* author of *Childhood and Society* (1950) and of major studies of Luther and Ghandi. He described psychosocial development in a human being in terms of eight stages: 1) trust vs. mistrust; 2) autonomy vs. doubt; 3) initiative vs. guilt; 4) industry vs. inferiority; 5) identity vs. role confusion; 6) intimacy vs. isolation; 7) generativity vs. self-absorption; and 8) integrity vs. despair.

erogenous zone An area of the body particularly susceptible to *erotic* arousal when stimulated, especially the oral, anal, and genital areas. Sometimes called erotogenic zone.

erotic Consciously or unconsciously invested with sexual feeling; sensually related.

erotomania See *-mania.*

erotomanic delusion See *delusional disorder.*

erythrophobia See under *phobia.*

ESP See *extrasensory perception.*

ethnology A science that concerns itself with the division of human beings into races and their origin, distribution, relations, and characteristics. See *cultural anthropology; social anthropology.*

ethology The scientific study of animal behavior; also the empirical study of human behavior.

etiology Causation, particularly with reference to disease.

euphoria An exaggerated feeling of physical and emotional well-being, usually of psychological origin. Also seen in *organic mental disorders* and in toxic and drug-induced states. See also *bipolar disorders.*

event-related potential Electrical activity produced by the brain in response to a sensory stimulus or associated with the execution of a motor, cognitive, or psychophysiological task. See also *electroencephalogram; evoked potential.*

evoked potential Electrical activity produced by the brain in response to any sensory stimulus; a more specific term than *event-related potential.* See also *electroencephalogram.*

excitement Agitation. See *catatonic behavior; psychomotor agitation.*

executive ego function A psychoanalytic term (see *psychoanalysis*) for the ego's management of the mental mechanisms in order to meet the needs of the organism. See also *ego.*

executive functioning Cognitive abilities such as planning, organizing, sequencing, and abstracting; may be seen in *dementia.*

exhibitionism One of the *paraphilias,* characterized by marked distress over, or acting on, urges to expose one's genitals to an unsuspecting stranger.

existential psychiatry (existentialism) A school of *psychiatry* evolved from orthodox psychoanalytic thought; stresses the way in which a person experiences the phenomenological world and takes responsibility for existence. Philosophically, it is *holistic* and self-deterministic in contrast to biologic or culturally deterministic points of view. See also *phenomenology* and OUTLINE OF SCHOOLS OF PSYCHIATRY.

existential psychotherapy A type of *psychotherapy* that emphasizes the person's inherent capacities to become healthy and fully functioning. It concentrates on the present, on achieving consciousness of life as being partially under one's control, on accepting responsibility for decisions, and on learning to tolerate *anxiety.*

exogenous psychoses *Organic mental disorders* originating outside the organism (e.g., disorders secondary to infection, intoxication, or trauma) or outside the neuropsychiatric "system" itself (e.g., hormonal, metabolic, or cardiovascular disorders). Contrast with *endogenous psychoses.*

experiential group A group whose main purpose is concerned with sharing whatever happens in a spontaneous fashion.

experiential therapy A generic term for a group of therapies that employ controlled or released emotion or "spiritual" experiences and power of conscious cognition and responsibility as the primary vehicles for inner growth and self-actualization. Included are 1) emotional-release therapies that are usually short-term and intense (encounter group therapy, gestalt therapy, primal scream therapy) and may emphasize body contact as the most direct vehicle for the release of emotional and muscular tensions (bioenergetic psychotherapy, rolfing); 2) emotional control therapies that focus on gaining greater control over the body through training (yoga, transcendental meditation); 3) religious and inspirational therapies (faith healing, Christian Science); and 4) cognitive-emotional therapies such as Ellis's rational-emotive psychotherapy (RET) and Glasser's reality therapy.

expert witness See LIST OF LEGAL TERMS.

explosive disorder, intermittent An *impulse control disorder* consisting of aggressive outbursts (e.g., assaultiveness or destruction of property) that are out of proportion to any evident stressors. Often the behavior is completely uncharacteristic of the person, who does not exhibit this behavior between episodes. In many cases, however, this aggressiveness comes out in less explosive ways between episodes.

explosive personality An *impulse control disorder* in which several episodes of serious outbursts of relatively unprovoked aggression lead to assault on others or the destruction of property. There is no demonstrable organic, epileptic, or any other *personality disorder* that might account for the behavior. Also called intermittent explosive personality.

expressed emotions The feelings that a family shows toward one of their members; specifically, over-involvement with and hostility and criticism directed toward a schizophrenic family member who lives with the family after discharge from a hospital.

expressive language disorder See *communication disorders.*

expressive writing disorder See *written expression, disorder of.*

extinction The weakening of a reinforced operant response as a result of ceasing *reinforcement.* See also *operant conditioning.* Also, the elimination of a conditioned response by repeated presentations of a conditioned stimulus without the unconditioned stimulus. See also *respondent conditioning.*

extrapyramidal syndrome A variety of signs and *symptoms,* including muscular rigidity, tremors, drooling, shuffling gait (*parkinsonism*); restlessness (*akathisia*); peculiar involuntary postures (*dystonia*); motor inertia (*akinesia*); and many other neurologic disturbances. Results from dysfunction of the *extrapyramidal system*. May occur as a reversible side effect of certain psychotropic drugs, particularly *phenothiazine derivatives*. See also *tardive dyskinesia* and LIST OF NEUROLOGIC DEFICITS.

extrapyramidal system The portion of the *central nervous system* responsible for coordinating and integrating various aspects of motor behavior or body movements. This is usually described in terms of cortical, *basal ganglia,* and midbrain levels of integration.

extrasensory perception (ESP) Perception without recourse to the conventional use of any of the five physical senses. See also *parapsychology; telepathy.*

extraversion A state in which attention and energies are largely directed outward from the self as opposed to inward toward the self, as in *introversion.*

eye tracking Various movements of the eyes (also called smooth pursuit eye movements) that enable the viewer to keep a moving target in focus. Eye-tracking abnormalities, such as jumpy extraneous eye movements that interfere with tracking, have been reported in 70% to 80% of patients with *schizophrenia* and in 45% to 50% of their first-degree relatives, but in only 6% of normal subjects.

F

facilitating environment A milieu that promotes the child's development of self-esteem and self-assertive ambitions. See *holding environment; mirroring.*

factitious disorders A group of disorders characterized by intentional production or feigning of physical
or psychological *symptoms* or signs related to a need
to assume the sick role rather than for obvious *secondary gains* such as economic support or obtaining
better care. The symptoms produced may be predominantly psychological, predominantly physical, or
a combination of both. An example is *Munchausen
syndrome.*

factor analysis A statistical technique that examines
population clusters to extract patterns of commonality.

failure to thrive A common problem in pediatrics in
which infants or young children show delayed physical growth, often with impaired social and motor
development. Nonorganic failure to thrive is thought
to be associated with lack of adequate emotional
nurturing. See *attachment disorder, reactive.*

faith healing See *experiential therapy.*

family therapy Treatment of more than one member
of a family in the same session. The treatment may be
supportive, directive, or interpretive. The assumption
is that a *mental disorder* in one member of a family
may be a manifestation of disorder in other members
and may affect interrelationships and functioning.

fantasy An imagined sequence of events or mental
images (e.g., daydreams) that serves to express *unconscious* conflicts, to gratify unconscious wishes, or
to prepare for anticipated future events.

FDA See *Food and Drug Administration.*

fear Unpleasant emotional and physiological response
to recognized sources of danger, to be distinguished
from *anxiety.* See also *phobia.*

feeblemindedness Obsolete term. See *mental retardation.*

feeding disorder of infancy or early childhood
Persistent failure to eat adequately, with loss of weight
or failure to gain weight, and not due to an associated

gastrointestinal or other *general medical condition.* In DSM-IV, feeding and eating disorders include *pica* and *rumination disorder.*

femaleness Anatomic and physiological features that relate to the female's procreative and nurturing capacities. See also *feminine.*

female orgasmic disorder One of the *orgasm disorders.*

female sexual arousal disorder One of the *sexual arousal disorders.* See *frigidity.*

female sexual desire disorder See *frigidity.*

feminine A set of sex-specific social role behaviors unrelated to procreative and nurturing biologic functions. See also *femaleness; gender identity; gender role.*

fetal alcohol syndrome A *congenital* disorder resulting from alcohol teratogenicity (i.e., the production, actual or potential, of pathological changes in the fetus, most frequently in the form of normal development of one or more organ systems; commonly referred to as birth defects), with the following possible dysmorphic categories: *central nervous system* dysfunction, birth deficiencies (such as low birth weight), facial abnormalities, and variable major and minor malformations. A safe level of alcohol use during pregnancy has not been established, and it is generally advisable for women to refrain from alcohol use during pregnancy.

fetishism One of the *paraphilias,* characterized by marked distress over, or acting on, sexual urges involving the use of nonliving objects (fetishes), such as underclothing, stockings, or boots.

fetishism, transvestic One of the *paraphilias,* characterized by marked distress over, or acting on, sexual urges involving cross-dressing, most frequently in a heterosexual male. The condition may occur with gender *dysphoria* as part of a *gender identity disorder,* but more commonly the transvestite has no desire to change his sex but wants only at a particular time to appear to be a female.

fixation The arrest of psychosocial development; may be considered pathological, depending on the degree of intensity.

flagellation See *masochism, sexual.*

flashback Hallucinogen persisting perception disorder or posthallucinogen perception disorder; reexperiencing, after ceasing the use of a hallucinogen, one or more of the perceptual *symptoms* that had been part of the hallucinatory experience while using the drug.

flexibilitas cerea See *cerea flexibilitas.*

flight of ideas A nearly continuous flow of accelerated speech with abrupt changes from one topic to another, usually based on understandable associations, distracting stimuli, or playing on words. When severe, however, this may lead to disorganized and incoherent speech. Flight of ideas is characteristic of *manic episodes,* but it may occur also in *organic mental disorders, schizophrenia,* other *psychoses,* and, rarely, acute reactions to stress.

flooding (implosion) A *behavior therapy* procedure for *phobias* and other problems involving maladaptive *anxiety,* in which anxiety producers are presented in intense forms, either in imagination or in real life. The presentations, which act as desensitizers, are continued until the stimuli no longer produce disabling anxiety.

focal psychotherapy *Brief psychotherapy* that concentrates on a central or core issue or a circumscribed area of conflict as the only or major object of intervention efforts. Focalization refers to the ability of the therapist and patient to agree on a psychodynamic target for the treatment.

folie à deux See *psychotic disorder, shared.*

follow-up examination Clinical assessment, often repeated at specific intervals following discharge from inpatient or outpatient treatment. Among its major purposes are to evaluate the need for adjustment of drug dosage, to detect signs of relapse, to measure improvement over time, and to identify (and, when possible, control) significant contributory factors to the maintenance or recurrence of *symptoms*.

Food and Drug Administration (FDA) One of a number of health administrations under the Assistant Secretary of Health (of the U.S. Department of Health and Human Services) to set standards for and license the sale of drugs and food substances, and in general to safeguard the public from the use of dangerous drugs and food substances.

forensic psychiatry A branch of *psychiatry* dealing with legal issues related to mental disorders. See also LIST OF LEGAL TERMS.

formal thought disorder An inexact term referring to a disturbance in the form of thinking rather than to abnormality of content. See *blocking; incoherence; loosening of associations; poverty of speech*.

formication The tactile *hallucination* or *illusion* that insects are crawling on the body or under the skin.

fragile X syndrome The most common form of inherited *mental retardation,* due to the abnormality of the X *chromosome.* The connection between the tip of the long arm of the abnormal chromosome and the rest of the chromosome is very slender and is easily broken, hence the term fragile X.

Clinical manifestations include moderate to severe mental retardation and a large head, long face, prominent ears, and, in affected males, large testicles. Some subjects with the abnormal gene are of normal intelligence but show one or more forms of *learning disability.* Many also have *attention-deficit/hyperactivity disorder (ADHD).*

fragmentation Separation into different parts, or preventing their integration, or detaching one or more parts from the rest. A fear of fragmentation of the personality, also known as disintegration anxiety, is often observed in patients whenever they are exposed to repetitions of earlier experiences that interfered with development of the self. This fear may be expressed as feelings of falling apart, as a loss of identity, or as a fear of impending loss of one's vitality and of psychological depletion.

free association In psychoanalytic therapy (see *psychoanalysis*), spontaneous, uncensored verbalization by the patient of whatever comes to mind.

free-floating anxiety Severe, generalized, persistent *anxiety* not specifically ascribed to a particular object or event and often a precursor of panic. See *generalized anxiety disorder*.

Freud, Anna (1895–1982) Austrian *psychoanalyst* and daughter of *Sigmund Freud,* noted for her contributions to the developmental theory of *psychoanalysis* and its applications to preventive work with children.

Freud, Sigmund (1856–1939) With Josef Breuer, he laid the foundation of *psychoanalysis* with the publication in 1893 of "On the Psychical Mechanism of Hysterical Phenomena: Preliminary Communication." This paper introduced Freud's seminal notion of psychological conflict. Freud's most famous work, *The Interpretation of Dreams* (1900), elucidated the nature of dreaming and primary process thinking and presented his initial observations concerning childhood sexuality, the oedipal conflict (see *Oedipus complex*), and the developmental roots of adult psychopathology.

Freud initially conceived of psychological conflict as existing between the *conscious,* self-preservative instinct of the *ego* and the repressed, mainly *unconscious* sexual instinct (libido)—the so-called topographic model of psychological functioning. In the early 1920s, Freud proposed a major revision of his theory with his formulation of the "structural model" of the mind that viewed the psyche as divided into the *ego, id,* and *superego*. This conceptual model set the stage for the elucidation of the psychological defenses and the subsequent important development of *ego psychology,* a central preoccupation of current psycho-analytic observation and theory.

frigidity Female sexual arousal disorder or female sexual desire disorder; it may consist of deficient or absent sexual fantasies and desire for sexual activity, aversion to and avoidance of genital sexual contact with a sexual partner, inability to attain or maintain the lubrication-swelling response of sexual excitement during sexual activity, or lack of a feeling of sexual excitement and pleasure during sexual activity.

frotteurism One of the *paraphilias,* consisting of recurrent, intense sexual urges involving touching and rubbing against a nonconsenting person; common sites in which such activities take place are crowded trains, buses, and elevators. Fondling the victim may be part of the condition and is called toucherism.

frozen watchfulness An alertness or even hypervigilance that is maintained despite an overall inhibition of motor activity that may include *mutism.*

fugue A *dissociative disorder* marked by sudden, unexpected travel away from one's customary environment, with inability to recall one's past and assumption of a new identity, which may be partial or complete.

functional In medicine, referring to changes in the way an organ system operates that are not attributed to known structural alterations. See also *functional disorder.*

functional disorder Abnormal performance or operation of an organ or organ system that is not a result of known changes in structure.

fusion The union and integration of the instincts and drives so that they complement each other and help the organism to deal effectively with both internal needs and external demands. *Aggression* can be used in the effective pursuit of the love object, for instance, and need not destroy object or self.

G

GABA Gamma-aminobutyric acid. A major inhibitory *neurotransmitter* in the brain, implicated in several psychiatric and neurologic conditions. See also *disinhibition*.

GAD *Generalized anxiety disorder.*

galvanic skin response (GSR) The change in the electrical resistance of the skin following stimulation; an easily measured variable widely used in experimental studies.

gambling, pathological An *impulse control disorder* whose pathological and maladaptive nature is suggested by the following: preoccupation with gambling; handicapping or planning the next venture with scheming to get money to gamble with; a need to gamble with more and more money in order to achieve the desired excitement; restlessness or irritability when attempting to reduce or stop gambling, or failure to stop; concealment of the extent of involvement in gambling from others; illegal activity used to finance gambling; or negative effects on significant relationships or career opportunities.

Ganser's syndrome Also called nonsense syndrome, syndrome of approximate answers, or prison psychosis; classified in DSM-IV as one of the *dissociative disorders*. It is characterized by giving deviously relevant or approximate answers to questions. Asked what a 25-cent piece is, the person says it is a dime. The syndrome is commonly associated with dissociative *amnesia* or *fugue*. Other symptoms may include disorientation, perceptual disturbances, and *conversion* symptoms. The syndrome is described most frequently in prison inmates for whom it may represent an attempt to gain leniency from prison or court officials.

gatekeeper In a *managed care* system, the person who decides what medical services a patient may have access to in nonemergency situations; often it is the *primary care physician,* but it may also be a non-physician case manager. See also *case management.*

gateway drugs Term coined by Robert Dupont, M.D., to refer to alcohol, cocaine, and marijuana, emphasizing that those three drugs are often the stepping-stones to more severe *addiction.*

Gault decision See LIST OF LEGAL TERMS.

gender identity (core gender identity) The inner sense of *maleness* or *femaleness* that identifies the person as being male, female, or ambivalent. Differentiation of gender identity usually takes place in infancy and early childhood and is reinforced by the hormonal changes of puberty. Gender identity is distinguished from sexual identity, which is biologically determined. See also *gender identity disorder; gender role.*

gender identity disorder One of the major groups of sexual and gender identity disorders, characterized by a strong and persistent identification with the opposite sex (cross-gender identification) and discomfort with one's assigned sex or a sense of inappropriateness in that gender role. Although onset is usually in childhood or adolescence, the disorder may not be presented clinically until adulthood. Manifestations include a repeated desire to be of the opposite sex, insistence that one has the typical feelings and reactions of the opposite sex, a belief that one was born the wrong sex, and transsexualism or preoccupation with one's primary and secondary sex characteristics in order to simulate the opposite sex.

gender role The image a person presents to others and to the self that declares him or her to be boy or girl, man or woman. Gender role is the public declaration of *gender identity,* but the two do not necessarily coincide.

general medical condition Any condition or disorder that is listed outside the mental disorders section of the *International Classification of Diseases (ICD).* The phrase is used in DSM-IV as a term of convenience only; it does not imply that there is any fundamental distinction between mental disorders and general medical conditions or that mental disorders are unrelated to physical or biological factors or processes.

general paralysis (general paresis) A form of tertiary neurosyphilis; a *general medical condition* occasionally associated with other neurologic signs of syphilitic involvement of the nervous system. Detectable with laboratory tests of the blood or spinal fluid. Formerly known as GPI (general paralysis of the insane), an obsolete term.

generalized anxiety disorder (GAD) Anxiety neurosis; characterized by unrealistic or excessive *anxiety,* apprehensive expectations, and worry about many life circumstances (e.g., academic, athletic, or social performance). A mother may worry endlessly about her child, who is in no danger. The worry is associated with *symptoms* such as trembling, muscle tension, restlessness, feelings of being smothered, lightheadedness, *insomnia,* exaggerated startle response, or difficulty in concentration. The worrying is difficult to control, and with associated symptoms, often social or occupational functioning is impaired.

When it occurs in childhood or adolescence, generalized anxiety disorder is termed *overanxious disor-*

der by some. Symptoms include multiple, unrealistic anxieties concerning the quality of one's performance in school, at work, or in sports, and of one's health or appearance, accompanied by the need to be reassured.

genes Located at various points along the *chromosomes,* genes are bits of *deoxyribonucleic acid* (DNA) that carry the hereditary code. It is estimated that the human has approximately 100,000 genes, known collectively as the genome.

genetic(s) In biology, pertaining to *genes* or to inherited characteristics. Also, in *psychiatry,* pertaining to the historical development of one's psychological attributes or disorders.

genetic counseling Advice given to a prospective parental couple regarding the inheritance of a pathological condition related to the couple's *genetic endowment.*

genetic endowment Inherited traits, potentials, and capacities.

genetic marker An abnormal DNA sequence that is associated with the presence of or vulnerability to a disease. More often than not, the abnormality is not the gene actually responsible for the disorder, but a DNA segment that remains physically close to the responsible gene and thus signals the presence of that gene. *Huntington's disease* is an example of the effects of the gene.

genetic viewpoint Psychoanalytic metapsychological hypothesis that is concerned with the origin and development of psychic phenomena in terms of how the past is contained in the present and why certain conflicts and adaptations were adopted by an individual.

genital phase See *psychosexual development.*

genotype The total set of *genes* present at the time of conception, producing the genetic constitution. See *phenotype.*

geriatric psychiatry Geropsychiatry; a subspecialty of *psychiatry* concerned with the psychological aspects of the *aging* process and *mental disorders* of the elderly.

geriatrics A branch of medicine dealing with the *aging* process and diseases of the aging human being.

gerontology The study of *aging*.

Gesell developmental schedules See TABLE OF PSY-CHOLOGICAL TESTS.

gestalt psychology A German school of *psychology* that emphasizes a total perceptual configuration and the interrelationships of its component parts. See also OUTLINE OF SCHOOLS OF PSYCHIATRY.

Gilles de la Tourette syndrome A genetically determined *syndrome* usually beginning in early childhood characterized by repetitive *tics,* other movement disorders, uncontrolled grunts, unintelligible sounds, and occasionally verbal obscenities. Also known as Tourette's disorder, part of the last name of Georges Gilles de la Tourette.

globus hystericus The disturbing sensation of a lump in the throat. See also *hysterical neurosis, conversion type* under *neurosis.*

glossolalia Gibberish-like speech or "speaking in tongues."

grand mal See *epilepsy.*

grandiose delusion See *delusional disorder.*

grandiose self One part of the *bipolar self* (see *Kohut*). The efforts of the child to elicit continuing praise from the parents by being perfect. The mother's generally positive responses to those efforts affirm the child's worth and promote the development of self-esteem and self-assertive ambitions, pursuit of goals, and enjoyment of physical and mental activities.

grandiosity Exaggerated belief or claims of one's importance or identity, often manifested by *delusions* of great wealth, power, or fame. See *bipolar disorders; mania.*

grief Normal, appropriate emotional response to an external and consciously recognized loss; it is usually time-limited and subsides gradually. To be distinguished from *depression.* See *mourning.*

group dynamics The interactions and interrelations among members of a therapy group and between members and the therapist. The effective use of group dynamics is essential in group treatment.

group practice A formal association of three or more physicians, or other health professionals, organized to provide a continuum of broader-based care than is usually provided by a single practitioner. Twenty-four-hour coverage by those within the group, different services, and different specialties make more services available, and management is less cumbersome and more patient-oriented than is possible in larger health care institutions.

group psychotherapy Application of psychotherapeutic techniques by a therapist who uses the emotional interactions of members of the group to help them get relief from distress and possibly modify their behavior. Typically, a group is composed of 4 to 12 persons who meet regularly with the therapist. See *group dynamics.*

groups See *group psychotherapy; sensitivity group.*

guardianship See LIST OF LEGAL TERMS.

guilt *Emotion* resulting from doing what one conceives of as wrong, thereby violating *superego* precepts; results in feelings of worthlessness and at times the need for punishment. See *shame.*

H

habeas corpus See LIST OF LEGAL TERMS.
habit disorder See *stereotypic movement disorder.*
hair pulling See *trichotillomania.*
halfway house A specialized residence for patients who do not require full hospitalization but who need an intermediate degree of domiciliary care before returning to independent community living.
hallucination A sensory perception in the absence of an actual external stimulus; to be distinguished from an *illusion,* which is a misperception or misinterpretation of an external stimulus. Hallucinations may involve any of the senses.

  auditory hallucination Perception of sound, most frequently of voices but sometimes of clicks or other noises.

  olfactory hallucination Perception of odor such as of burning rubber or decaying fish.

  somatic hallucination Perception of a physical sensation within the body such as a feeling of electricity running through one's body.

  tactile hallucination Perception of being touched or of something being under one's skin such as the sensation of pins being stuck into one's finger. The sensation of something crawling under one's skin is called *formication;* it occurs most frequently in *alcohol withdrawal syndrome* and in *cocaine* withdrawal.

  visual hallucination Perception of an image such as people (formed) or a flash of light (unformed).

hallucinogen A chemical agent that produces *hallucinations.* The term is used synonymously with *psychotomimetic.*

hallucinogen use disorders In DSM-IV, this group includes hallucinogen dependence, hallucinogen abuse, hallucinogen intoxication, hallucinogen persisting perception disorder (flashbacks), hallucinogen delirium, hallucinogen psychotic disorder, hallucinogen mood disorder, and hallucinogen anxiety disorder.

hallucinosis A condition in which the patient hallucinates in a state of clear consciousness, as in *alcohol hallucinosis.*

DSM-IV classifies what was "organic" hallucinosis on the basis of whether or not *reality testing* about the hallucinatory experiences is intact. In patients whose reality testing is impaired, hallucinosis is termed substance-induced (e.g., alcohol) psychotic disorder with hallucinations. In patients whose reality testing is intact, hallucinosis is termed substance-induced intoxication (or withdrawal) with perceptual disturbance.

haloperidol See TABLE OF DRUGS USED IN PSYCHIATRY.

Halstead-Reitan See TABLE OF PSYCHOLOGICAL TESTS.

Health and Human Services A federal department established in 1953 as the U.S. Department of Health, Education, and Welfare to supervise and coordinate the following agencies: *Food and Drug Administration;* Office of Human Development; Public Health Service; Social Security Administration; *Substance Abuse and Mental Health Services Administration; National Institutes of Health;* Centers for Disease Control; Health Care Financing Administration; Office of Children, Youth and Families; and Office of Smoking and Health. In 1979, a separate Department of Education was established, and the remaining agencies became the Department of Health and Human Services.

health care proxy See *living will.*

health maintenance organization (HMO) A form of *group practice* by physicians and supporting personnel to provide comprehensive health services to an enrolled group of subscribers who pay a fixed premium (*capitation* fee) to belong. Emphasis is on maintaining the health of the enrollees as well as treating their illnesses. HMOs must include psychiatric benefits to receive federal support.

hebephrenic schizophrenia See *schizophrenia.*

hedonism Pleasure-seeking behavior. Contrast with *anhedonia.*

helplessness Actual or self-perceived inability to act on one's own behalf; inefficiency in making an impact on one's environment to create change.

heroin An illicit (in the United States) opioid synthesized from morphine. Heroin, a white or brown powder, is injected intravenously and is the most commonly abused narcotic.

heterogeneity Dissimilarity in the genotypic structure of individuals originating through sexual reproduction.

HEW Health, Education, and Welfare; see *Health and Human Services.*

5-HIAA (5-hydroxyindoleacetic acid) A major metabolite of *serotonin,* a *biogenic amine* found in the brain and other organs. Functional deficits of serotonin in the *central nervous system* have been implicated in certain types of major *mood disorders,* and particularly in *suicide* and impulsivity.

high-risk behavior Actions that put one in danger or render one vulnerable to harmful consequences. Needle sharing by addicts, for example, is high-risk behavior because of the likelihood of transmission of HIV or other pathogens.

hippocampus Olfactory brain; a sea-horse–shaped structure located within the brain that is an important part of the *limbic system.* The hippocampus is involved in some aspects of memory, in the control of the autonomic functions, and in emotional expression.

histrionic See *personality disorder.*

HIV dementia Also, AIDS dementia complex (ADC); a rapidly progressive subcortical *dementia* characterized by 1) cognitive deficits such as inattentiveness, impaired concentration and problem solving, forgetfulness, and impaired reading; 2) motor abnormalities such as tremors, slurred speech, *ataxia,* and generalized *hyperreflexia;* and 3) behavioral changes such as sluggishness and social withdrawal. *CT* and *MRI* usually indicate brain atrophy along with an enlargement of the ventricles.

HIV dementia characteristically begins with impaired concentration and mild memory loss. Over a period of several weeks or months, the condition progresses to severe global cognitive impairment.

HIV meningitis An acute aseptic meningitis that occurs soon after infection with the virus. *Symptoms,* which are usually mild and self-limited, include headache, fever, painful sensitivity to light, and cranial neuropathy. The symptoms typically disappear in 1 to 4 weeks.

Cryptococcal meningitis is a more serious form of meningitis that occurs in HIV-infected persons as a result of infection with the common soil fungus, Cryptococcus neoformans. Symptoms include headache, stiff neck, fever, and painful sensitivity to light.

holding environment A responsive, nurturing milieu for the developing child, including physical holding as well as the mother's or primary caregiver's preoccupation with the child and her ability to soothe, comfort, and reduce the tension in her infant. Ideally, the mother reflects back the child's worth and value and in other ways responds appropriately to his or her needs. Lack of such responsivity is often termed *empathic failure.*

In the psychotherapeutic (see *psychotherapy*) relationship, holding environment refers to a therapeutic ambiance or setting that permits the patient to experience safety, thereby facilitating psychotherapeutic work.

holism An approach to the study of the individual in totality, rather than as an aggregate of separate physiological, psychological, and social characteristics.

homeostasis Self-regulating biological and psychological processes that maintain the stability and equilibrium of the organism.

homosexual panic An acute and severe attack of *anxiety* based on *unconscious* conflicts involving *gender identity;* Kempf's disease.

homosexuality A primary *erotic* attraction to others of the same sex that is increasingly viewed as a constitutional, probably largely inherited trait. Overt homosexual behavior may be inhibited, delayed, or otherwise modified because of family or peer pressure, social bias, or internal conflict caused by the internalization of social prejudice.

homosexuality, ego-dystonic A sustained pattern of overt homosexual arousal that is a source of distress. When DSM-III was revised in 1987, ego-dystonic homosexuality was deleted as a diagnostic entity because "almost all people who are homosexual first go through a phase in which their homosexuality is ego dystonic" (Appendix, DSM-III-R). This category is not included in DSM-IV.

homovanillic acid (HVA) A principal metabolite of *dopamine,* a *catecholamine* found in the brain and other organs.

hormone A discrete chemical substance secreted into the body fluids by an endocrine gland, which has a specific effect on the activities of other organs. See also *neurohormone.*

Horney, Karen (1885–1952) German *psychoanalyst* who emigrated to the United States in 1932, departed from orthodox Freudian thought and founded her own school, emphasizing cultural factors underlying *neurosis*. See OUTLINE OF SCHOOLS OF PSYCHIATRY.

Hospital and Community Psychiatry An interdisciplinary monthly journal of the *American Psychiatric Association.*

hostility Actual or threatened aggressive contact, destructive in intent.

hotline Telephone assistance service for crisis intervention, usually focused on topics such as alcoholic binges, *suicide,* drugs, and runaways.

humiliation Sense of disgrace and shame often experienced in *depression.*

Huntington's disease (chorea) A rare hereditary and progressive degenerative disease of the *central nervous system* transmitted as an autosomal dominant trait. Onset is typically in middle adult life with involuntary movements of the face, hands, and shoulders. These movements become more pronounced and often result in a massive jerkiness of the limbs, facial muscles, and diaphragm. Progressive *dementia* typically parallels the movement disorder and the person is incapable of doing anything. *Psychosis* may develop, most commonly *depression* that varies in degree (ill-sustained).

hyperactivity Excessive motor activity that may be purposeful or aimless; movements and utterances are usually more rapid than normal. Hyperactivity is a prominent feature of attention-deficit disorder, so much so that in DSM-IV the latter is called *attention-deficit/hyperactivity disorder (ADHD).*

hyperactivity disorder See *attention-deficit/hyperactivity disorder.*

hyperacusis Inordinate sensitivity to sounds; it may be on an emotional or an organic basis.

hyperkinetic disorder See *attention-deficit/hyperactivity disorder.*

hyperreflexia Overactive or overresponsive reflexes, such as the ankle jerk or the knee jerk, suggestive of upper motor neuron disease and lessening or loss of control ordinarily exerted by higher brain centers of lower neural pathways (*disinhibition*).

hypersomnia A *dyssomnia* consisting of prolonged or daytime *sleep* episodes occurring almost daily. The hypersomnia is called primary if it is not related to another *mental disorder*, if it is not substance induced, and if it is not due to a *general medical condition*.

hypertensive crisis Sudden and sometimes fatal rise in blood pressure; it may occur as a result of combining *monoamine oxidase inhibitors* with *tyramine* in food or with other sympathomimetic substances (e.g., cough remedies and nose drops).

hyperventilation Overbreathing sometimes associated with *anxiety* and marked by reduction of blood carbon dioxide, producing complaints of light-headedness, faintness, tingling of the extremities, palpitations, and respiratory distress.

hypesthesia Diminished sensitivity to tactile stimuli.

hypnagogic Referring to the semiconscious state immediately preceding sleep; may include *hallucinations* that are of no pathological significance.

hypnopompic Referring to the state immediately preceding awakening; may include *hallucinations* that are of no pathological significance.

hypnosis A state of decreased general awareness with heightened attention to a constricted or localized area of stimulation, such as repetitive suggestions by another person (the hypnotist) involving consciousness, memory, anesthesia, or paralysis. The state usually is associated with the feeling that the subject is behaving nonvolitionally even though aware of what the behavior is. Factors determining the subject's responsivity include the nature of the preexisting relationship with the hypnotist; prior expectations, beliefs, and motivations concerning hypnosis; and, most important, characterological and individual differences.

hypnotic Any agent that induces *sleep*. Although *sedatives, narcotics,* or *anxiolytics* in sufficient dosage may produce sleep as an incidental effect, the term hypnotic is appropriately reserved for drugs employed primarily to produce sleep.

hypnotic use disorder See *sedative/hypnotic/anxiolytic use disorders.*

hypoactive sexual desire disorder See *sexual desire disorders.*

hypochondriasis One of the *somatoform disorders,* characterized by persisting worry about health or fear of having some disease despite appropriate medical reassurance and lack of findings on physical or laboratory examination. Fear of contracting a disease is considered to be a *phobia* rather than hypochondriasis.

hypoglycemia Abnormally low level of blood sugar. See *insulin coma treatment.*

hypomania A psychopathological state and abnormality of *mood* falling somewhere between normal *euphoria* and *mania.* It is characterized by unrealistic optimism, pressure of speech and activity, and a decreased need for *sleep.* Some people show increased creativity during hypomanic states, whereas others show poor judgment, irritability, and irascibility. See *bipolar disorders.*

hypomanic episode Characteristics are the same as in a *manic episode* but not so severe as to cause marked impairment in social or occupational functioning or to require hospitalization, even though the *mood* change is clearly different from the subject's usual non-depressed mood and is observable to others. See *bipolar disorders.*

hypothalamus The complex brain structure composed of many nuclei with various functions. It is the head ganglion of the *autonomic nervous system* and is involved in the control of heat regulation; heart rate, blood pressure, and respiration; sexual activity; water, fat, and carbohydrate metabolism; digestion, appetite, and body weight; wakefulness; fight or flight response; and rage.

hypoventilation, central aveolar *Sleep apnea.* See *breathing-related sleep disorder.*

hysterical personality See *histrionic* under *personality disorder.*

hysterics Lay term for uncontrollable emotional outbursts.

I

---

iatrogenic illness A disorder precipitated, aggravated, or induced by the physician's attitude, examination, comments, or treatment.

ICD-9 The 9th revision of the *International Classification of Diseases.*

ICD-10 The 10th revision of the *International Classification of Diseases.*

id In Freudian theory (see *Freud*), the part of the personality that is the *unconscious* source of unstructured desires and drives. See also *ego; superego.*

idealization A mental mechanism in which the person attributes exaggeratedly positive qualities to the self or others.

idealized parental imago In *Kohut's self psychology,* the archaic selfobject to which the child, as is appropriate for his or her phase of development, needs to look up, admire, and feel attached. When development is successful, it becomes transformed into internalized values and ideals that are soothing, drive-channeling structures that maintain and restore internal balance. The idealized parental imago is one pole of the *bipolar self;* the other pole is the *grandiose self.*

idealizing transference See *transference, selfobject.*

ideas of reference Incorrect interpretations of casual incidents and external events as having direct reference to oneself. May reach sufficient intensity to constitute *delusions.*

idée fixe Fixed idea. Used in *psychiatry* to describe a *compulsive* drive, an obsessive idea, or a *delusion.*

identification A *defense mechanism,* operating unconsciously, by which one patterns oneself after some other person. Identification plays a major role in the development of one's personality and specifically of the *superego.* To be differentiated from imitation or role modeling, which is a *conscious* process.

identity The sense of self and unity of personality over time; one element of identity is *gender identity.* Identity disturbances are seen in identity disorder, borderline *personality disorder,* and *schizophrenia.*

identity crisis A loss of the sense of the sameness and historical continuity of one's self and an inability to accept or adopt the role one perceives as being expected by society. This is often expressed by isolation, withdrawal, extremism, rebelliousness, and negativity, and is typically triggered by a sudden increase in the strength of instinctual *drives* in a milieu of rapid social evolution and technological change. See *psychosocial development.*

identity disorder, dissociative See *multiple personality disorder.*

identity disorder, gender See *gender identity disorder.*

identity problem This term is applied to adolescents who are in the process of detaching themselves from their families and parental value systems in an attempt to establish their own independent identities.

idiopathic Of unknown cause.

idiot savant A person with gross *mental retardation* who nonetheless is capable of performing certain remarkable feats in sharply circumscribed intellectual areas, such as calendar calculation or puzzle solving.

illusion A misperception of a real external stimulus. Example: the rustling of leaves is heard as the sound of voices. Contrast with *hallucination.*

imago A term used by *Jung* for an *unconscious* mental image, usually an *idealization,* of an important person in one's early history.

immediate memory The recall of perceived material within a period of 30 seconds to 25 minutes after presentation.

implosion See *flooding.*

impotence The inability to achieve or maintain a penile erection of sufficient quality to engage in successful sexual intercourse; male erectile disorder. Two types are described by Masters and Johnson: in primary impotence, there has never been a successful sexual coupling; in secondary impotence, failure occurs following at least one successful union. Compare with *orgasmic dysfunction.* See *sexual arousal disorders.*

impotence, ejaculatory See *orgasm disorders.*

impotence, erectile See *sexual arousal disorders.*

imprinting A term in *ethology* referring to a process similar to rapid learning or behavioral patterning that occurs at critical points in very early stages of animal development. The extent to which imprinting occurs in human development has not been established.

impulse A desire or propensity to act in a certain way, typically in order to ease tension or gain pleasure.

impulse control disorders Failing to resist an *impulse,* drive, or temptation to perform some act that is harmful to oneself or to others. The impulse may be resisted consciously, but it is consonant with the person's immediate, *conscious* wish. The act may be premeditated or unplanned. The person may display regret or guilt for the action or its consequenses. In DSM-IV, this category includes *pathological gambling, kleptomania, pyromania,* intermittent explosive disorder, and *trichotillomania.*

inappropriate affect A display of *emotion* that is out of harmony with reality or with the verbal or intellectual content that it accompanies. See *affect.*

incest Sexual activity between close blood relatives, such as father-daughter, mother-son, or between siblings.

incidence The frequency of onset or occurrence of a disorder. See LIST OF RESEARCH TERMS.

incoherence Lacking in unity or consistency; often applied to speech or thinking that is not understandable owing to any of the following: lack of logical connection between words or phrases; excessive use of incomplete sentences; many irrelevancies or abrupt changes in subject matter; idiosyncratic word usage; or distorted grammar. See also *loosening of associations.*

incompetency Lack of the capacity to understand the nature of, to assess adequately, or to manage effectively a specified transaction or situation that the ordinary person could reasonably be expected to handle. As used in the law, the term refers primarily to *cognitive* defects that interfere with judgment.

incorporation A primitive *defense mechanism,* operating unconsciously, in which the psychic representation of a person, or parts of the person, is figuratively ingested. See *introjection.*

indigenous worker See *caregiver.*

individual psychology A system of psychiatric theory, research, and therapy developed by Alfred *Adler* that stresses *compensation* and *overcompensation* for inferiority feelings (inferiority *complex*).

individuation A process of *differentiation,* the end result of which is development of the individual personality that is separate and distinct from all others.

indoleamine One of a group of *biogenic amines* (e.g., *serotonin*) that contains a five-membered, nitrogen-containing indole ring and an *amine* group within its chemical structure.

indoles A group of biogenic compounds that include *indoleamines.*

induced factitious symptoms See *factitious disorders.*

induced psychotic disorder See *psychotic disorder, shared.*

industrial psychiatry See *occupational psychiatry.*

infancy, childhood, and adolescence disorders In DSM-IV, the full title for this section is "Disorders Usually First Diagnosed During Infancy, Childhood, or Adolescence." Included are mental *retardation, learning disorders, motor skills disorder, pervasive developmental disorders, disruptive behavior and attention-deficit disorders, feeding and eating disorders of infancy or early childhood, tic disorders, communication disorders, elimination disorders,* and others (including *separation anxiety disorder,* selective *mutism,* reactive *attachment disorder,* and *stereotypic movement disorder*).

infant psychiatry An aspect of *child and adolescent psychiatry* that deals with the diagnosis, treatment, and prevention of maladaptive psychological functioning in the very young.

infantile autism See *autism.*

infantilism See *masochism, sexual* for one form of infantilism.

inferiority complex See *individual psychology.*

infibulation See *masochism, sexual.*

informed consent Permission by the patient for a medical procedure based on understanding the nature of the procedure, the risks involved, the consequences of withholding permission, and alternative procedures. See LIST OF LEGAL TERMS.

infradian rhythms See *biological rhythms.*

inhalant use disorders In DSM-IV, this group includes inhalant dependence, inhalant abuse, inhalant intoxicaton, inhalant delirium, inhalant persisting dementia, inhalant psychotic disorder with delusions or hallucinations, inhalant mood disorder, and inhalant anxiety disorder.

inhibited orgasm See *orgasm disorders.*

inhibition Behavioral evidence of an *unconscious* defense against forbidden instinctual drives (see *instinct*); may interfere with or restrict specific activities.

insane Obsolete term referring to the state of having a *mental disorder.*

insanity An obsolete term for *psychosis.* Still used, however, in strictly legal contexts such as insanity defense.

insanity defense See LIST OF LEGAL TERMS.

insecurity A feeling of helplessness against *anxiety* arising from uncertainty about one's goals, ideals, abilities, and relationships.

insight Self-understanding; the extent of a person's understanding of the origin, nature, and mechanisms of his or her maladaptive attitudes and behavior.

insomnia A *dyssomnia* consisting of difficulty initiating or maintaining *sleep,* or of nonrestorative sleep (i.e., sleep is adequate in amount but unrefreshing), associated with daytime fatigue or impaired daytime functioning. The insomnia is called primary if it is not related to another mental disorder, if it is not substance induced, and if it is not due to a *general medical condition.*

instinct An inborn *drive*. The primary human instincts include self-preservation, sexuality, and—according to some proponents—the death instinct, of which *aggression* is one manifestation.

institutionalization Long-term placement of an individual into a hospital, nursing home, residential center, or other facility where independent living is restricted in varying degrees.

insulin coma treatment Injection of insulin in sufficient quantity to produce profound *hypoglycemia* (low blood sugar) resulting in *coma*. First used in 1933 in the treatment of *schizophrenia*, it is rarely used today.

intake The initial interview between a patient and a member of a psychiatric team in a mental health facility.

integration The useful organization and incorporation of both new and old data, experience, and emotional capacities into the *personality*. Also refers to the organization and amalgamation of functions at various levels of *psychosexual development*.

intellectualization A mental mechanism in which the person engages in excessive abstract thinking to avoid confrontation with conflicts or disturbing feelings.

intelligence Capacity to learn and to utilize appropriately what one has learned. May be affected by *emotions*.

intelligence quotient (IQ) A numerical rating determined through psychological testing that indicates the approximate relationship of a person's mental age (MA) to chronological age (CA). Expressed mathematically as IQ = [MA ÷ CA] x 100. See also TABLE OF PSYCHOLOGICAL TESTS.

interictal behavior syndrome Sometimes termed temporal lobe epileptic personality, it is manifested as a change in personality in three areas: 1) sexuality such as sexual *paraphilias*, conflicts over sexual preference, or hyposexuality; 2) aggressivity such as aggressive actions, moral indignation, or plans for retaliation for imagined slights; and 3) emotions and intellect such as *compulsive* writing or drawing (often related to religious or philosophical speculations), preoccupation with details, and a clinging quality in relations with others. See *epilepsy.*

intermittent explosive disorder See *explosive disorder, intermittent.*

internal capsule See *basal ganglia.*

International Classification of Diseases (ICD) The official list of disease categories issued by the World Health Organization; subscribed to by all member nations, who may assign their own terms to each ICD category. The ICDA (International Classification of Diseases, U.S. Public Health Service adaptation) represents the official list of diagnostic terms to be used for each ICD category in the United States.

internship The first year of graduate medical education, which ordinarily is integrated into a full residency training program in a designated specialty. Currently, PGY-1 (first postgraduate training year) tends to be the preferred term.

interpersonal psychotherapy (IPT) A form of brief (12 to 15 weeks) *psychotherapy* originally developed by Klerman, Weissman, and colleagues for the treatment of *depression* in which the focus is on four interpersonal problem areas often associated with its onset: grief, role disputes, role transitions, and interpersonal deficits. The focus is on current problems, important social relations, self-evaluation by the patient with assessment of his or her current situation, and clarification and modification of maladaptive perceptions and current interpersonal relationships. A procedural manual specifies the concept, techniques, and strategies of interpersonal therapy.

interpersonal skills Effective adaptive behavior in relation to other persons.

interpretation The process by which the therapist brings the patient to an understanding of a particular aspect of the problems or behavior.

intoxication Poisoning; especially the acute effects of overdosage with chemical substances. Characteristically, intoxication with substances of abuse produces behavioral or psychological changes because of their effects on the *central nervous system*. Such changes may be expressed as belligerence, differences in *mood,* or impaired judgment.

> **alcohol** Typical *symptoms* include maladaptive behavioral changes such as inappropriate aggressive or sexual behavior, *lability* of mood, and impaired judgment. The accompanying physical signs include slurred speech, incoordination, unsteady gait, and flushed face.

> **amphetamine** Typical *symptoms* include maladaptive psychological or behavioral changes such as *euphoria* with enhanced vigor and alertness or grandiosity; affective blunting with fatigue or sadness; changes in sociability ranging from gregariousness to social withdrawal; hypervigilance and sensitivity, sometimes leading to fighting; *anxiety,* tension, or anger; stereotyped, repetitive behavior; and impaired judgment. Perceptual disturbances may also occur. Accompanying physical signs may include very rapid or very slow heartbeat, elevated or lowered blood pressure, perspiration or chills, nausea, evidence of weight loss, muscular weakness, chest pain, and confusion.

> **caffeine** Consumption of caffeine, generally more than 250 mg, produces signs including restlessness, nervousness, excitement, *insomnia,* flushed face, muscle twitching, rambling speech, and *psychomotor agitation.*

cannabis Within 2 hours of cannabis use, the subject shows maladaptive behavioral or psychological changes such as impaired motor coordination, *euphoria, anxiety,* suspiciousness, sensation of slowed time, impaired judgment, and social withdrawal. Physical signs may include increased appetite, dry mouth, and very rapid heartbeat.

cocaine Signs and *symptoms* are the same as in *amphetamine intoxication* (see above).

hallucinogen The *syndrome* includes maladaptive behavioral or psychological changes such as marked anxiety or *depression,* fear of losing one's mind, paranoid ideation, and impaired judgment. Also, perceptual changes such as intensified perceptions, *illusions, hallucinations, derealization,* and *depersonalization* occur in a state of full wakefulness. Some physical signs include sweating, very rapid heartbeat, blurring of vision, tremors, and incoordination.

inhalant Recent use or short-term, high-dose exposure to volatile inhalants often leads to maladaptive behavioral or psychological changes such as belligerence, assaultiveness, apathy, and impaired judgment. The accompanying physical signs include dizziness, incoordination, slurred speech, unsteady gait, euphoria, lethargy, *psychomotor retardation,* and blurred vision.

opioid Signs of this *syndrome* include initial euphoria followed by apathy, psychomotor agitation or retardation, and impaired judgment. Diminished pupil size in the eyes, drowsiness, slurred speech, and impairment in attention or memory are some of the physical indicators.

phencyclidine Recent use of phencyclidine or a related substance may induce belligerence, assaultiveness, impulsiveness, unpredictability, and impaired judgment. The physical signs may include hypertension or a very rapid heartbeat, numbness or diminished responsiveness to pain, *ataxia,* muscle rigidity, or seizures.

sedative Effects of sedative intoxication are similar to those of *alcohol intoxication*. Signs include inappropriate sexual or aggressive behavior, swings in mood, and impaired judgment. Associated physical signs may include slurred speech, incoordination, unsteady gait, and impairment in attention or memory.

intrapsychic Taking place within the *psyche* or mind.

intrapsychic conflict See *conflict.*

intravenous (IV) Within or into the veins.

introjection A *defense mechanism,* operating unconsciously (see *unconscious*), whereby loved or hated external objects are symbolically absorbed within oneself. The converse of *projection.* May serve as a defense against *conscious* recognition of intolerable hostile impulses. For example, in severe *depression,* the individual may unconsciously direct unacceptable hatred or *aggression* toward herself or himself. Related to the more primitive *fantasy* of oral *incorporation.*

introspection Self-observation; examination of one's feelings, often as a result of *psychotherapy.*

introversion Preoccupation with oneself and accompanying reduction of interest in the outside world. Contrast to *extraversion.*

involutional melancholia A term formerly used to describe an agitated *depression* in a person of *climacteric* age. Currently, such patients are not distinguished from depressed patients of other age groups.

isolation A *defense mechanism* operating unconsciously (see *unconscious*) central to obsessive-compulsive phenomena in which the *affect* is detached from an idea and rendered unconscious, leaving the *conscious* idea colorless and emotionally neutral.

IQ *Intelligence quotient.*
ITP *Interpersonal psychotherapy.*

— **J** —

Jacksonian epilepsy See *epilepsy.*
James, William (1842–1910) American philosopher and *psychologist,* James graduated from Harvard Medical School but never practiced medicine. However, as Professor of Psychology and Philosophy at Harvard College and founder of the Laboratory of Experimental Psychology (where Gertrude Stein worked as a graduate student), he made major contributions to the understanding of *psychopathology* through his extensive studies, writing, and lectures dealing with mental *dissociation* and *unconscious* mental phenomena.
Janet, Pierre (1859–1947) French *psychiatrist* who first provided solid empirical evidence for the existence of *unconscious* (subconscious) mental processes. He advanced the concept of mental *dissociation* and formulated theories of hysterical symptoms and dissociative conditions that were based on the concept of constitutional deficits in psychological energy and functioning rather than on the concept of psychological conflict, which characterized *Freud's* developing psychoanalytic theoretical framework.
jealousy delusion See *delusional disorder.*
Joint Commission on Accreditation of Healthcare Organizations (JCAHO) Formerly Joint Commission on Accreditation of Hospitals (JCAH); the agency that surveys hospitals and other health facilities and programs and certifies that they have met the standards set by the Joint Commission. See *accreditation.*

Jones, Ernest (1879–1958) English pathologist and, later, *psychoanalyst* who was an early pupil of *Freud* and his principal biographer. Jones introduced *psychoanalysis* to the English-speaking world through his lectures on the subject.

judgment Mental act of comparing choices between a given set of values in order to select a course of action.

Jung, Carl Gustav (1875–1961) Swiss *psychoanalyst;* founder of the school of *analytic psychology.* See also *anima; imago; persona;* and OUTLINE OF SCHOOLS OF PSYCHIATRY.

K

kinesics The study of body posture, movement, and facial expressions.

Kirkbride, Thomas S. (1809–1883) American *psychiatrist,* who was one of the founders of the *American Psychiatric Association.* Noted for his pioneering contributions to mental hospital design.

Klein, Melanie (1882–1960) Austrian-born British pioneer in the *psychoanalysis* of children. Noted for her work on early childhood development, particularly infantile aggression and the origins of the *superego* in early infancy. She is considered the founder of British object-relations theory. See also OUTLINE OF SCHOOLS OF PSYCHIATRY.

Kleine-Levin syndrome Periodic episodes of *hypersomnia;* first appears in *adolescence,* usually in boys, and is accompanied by bulimia. It is not classified as either an eating disorder or a sleep disorder. It is considered a neurologic *syndrome* and is believed to reflect a frontal lobe or hypothalamic disturbance.

kleptomania An *impulse control disorder* consisting of episodes of stealing objects that are not needed for personal use or for their monetary value. As in other disorders of impulse control, an increasing sense of tension or affective arousal immediately precedes the action, and the completion of the action brings a sense of pleasure or relief.

Klinefelter's syndrome Chromosomal defect in males in which there is an extra X *chromosome;* manifestations may include underdeveloped testes, physical feminization, sterility, and *mental retardation.*

klismaphilia One of the *paraphilias,* characterized by marked distress over, or acting on, sexual urges involving enemas.

Klüver-Bucy syndrome A syndrome following bilateral temporal lobe removal consisting of loss of recognition of people, loss of fear, rage reactions, hypersexuality, excessive oral behavior, memory defect, and overreaction to visual stimuli.

Kohut, Heinz (1913–1981) An Austrian-born American *psychoanalyst* who received his medical degree from the University of Vienna and then trained in *neurology* and *psychiatry* at the University of Chicago. He developed concepts and theories of *self psychology.* See *bipolar self; empathic failure; grandiose self; idealized parental imago.*

koro See *culture-specific syndromes.*

Korsakoff's syndrome A disease associated with chronic *alcoholism,* resulting from a deficiency of vitamin B_1. Patients sustain damage to part of the thalamus and cerebellum. *Symptoms* include inflammation of nerves, muttering *delirium, insomnia, illusions,* and *hallucinations.* See *alcohol psychosis; Wernicke-Korsakoff syndrome.*

Kraepelin, Emil (1856–1926) German *psychiatrist* who developed an extensive systematic classification of mental illnesses. One of the first to delineate the concept of *dementia praecox* (or *schizophrenia*). See also *descriptive psychiatry.*

Krafft-Ebing, Richard von (1840–1902) German *neuropsychiatrist* and student of sexual pathology, remembered for his now classic *Psychopathia Sexualis,* a pioneering study of sexual aberrations, published in 1886.

L

la belle indifférence Literally, "beautiful indifference." Seen in certain patients with *conversion* disorders who show an inappropriate lack of concern about their disabilities. See *hysterical neurosis, conversion type,* under *neurosis.* See also *Janet.*

labile Rapidly shifting (as applied to *emotions*); unstable.

lability of affect See *affect.*

lacrimation Tearing; it may be a significant *symptom* in opioid withdrawal.

language disorder See *communication disorders.*

lapsus linguae A slip of the tongue due to *unconscious* factors.

latah See *culture-specific syndromes.*

late luteal phase dysphoric disorder See *premenstrual dysphoric disorder.*

latency period See *psychosexual development.*

latent content The hidden (i.e., *unconscious*) meaning of thoughts or actions, especially in dreams or fantasies. In dreams, it is expressed in distorted, disguised, condensed, and symbolic form.

learned helplessness A condition in which a person attempts to establish and maintain contact with another by adopting a helpless, powerless stance.

learning disability A *syndrome* affecting school-age children of normal or above-normal intelligence characterized by specific difficulties in learning to read (*dyslexia,* word-blindness), write (dysgraphia), and calculate (dyscalculia). The disorder is believed to be related to slow developmental progression of perceptual motor skills. See *minimal brain dysfunction.*

learning disorders See *academic skills disorders.*

lesbian Homosexual woman. See *homosexuality.*

lethality scale Set of criteria used to predict *suicide.*

lethologica Temporary inability to remember a proper noun or name.

liaison nursing Consultation by clinical specialists in psychiatric nursing to nursing colleagues on issues of patient management in medical-surgical, parent-child, or geriatric settings. See also *psychiatric nurse.*

liaison psychiatry See *consultation-liaison psychiatry.*

libido The psychic *drive* or energy usually associated with the sexual *instinct.* (Sexual is used here in the broad sense to include pleasure and love-object seeking.)

limbic system Visceral brain; a group of brain structures—including the *amygdala, hippocampus,* septum, cingulate gyrus, and subcallosal gyrus—that work to help regulate *emotion,* memory, and certain aspects of movement.

lithium carbonate An alkali metal, the salt of which is used in the treatment of acute *mania* and as a maintenance medication to help reduce the duration, intensity, and frequency of recurrent affective episodes, especially in *bipolar disorders.*

living will One type of advanced directive; a competent person gives instructions for medical care, indicating the kind of care that will be consented to or refused. See LIST OF LEGAL TERMS.

lobotomy A type of *psychosurgery* in which one or more nerve tracts in the cerebrum are severed. This procedure is now rarely used in the United States except for intractable *obsessive-compulsive disorder.*

locus coeruleus A small area in the brain stem containing *norepinephrine* neurons that is considered to be a key brain center for *anxiety* and *fear.*

logorrhea Uncontrollable, excessive talking.

logotherapy A form of *existential psychotherapy* associated with the name of Viktor Frankl. See OUTLINE OF SCHOOLS OF PSYCHIATRY.

long-term memory The final phase of memory in which information storage may last from hours to a lifetime. Contrast with *immediate memory.*

loosening of associations A disturbance of thinking shown by speech in which ideas shift from one subject to another that is unrelated or minimally related to the first. Statements that lack a meaningful relationship may be juxtaposed, or speech may shift suddenly from one frame of reference to another. The speaker gives no indication of being aware of the disconnectedness, contradictions, or illogicality of speech. See also *incoherence.*

loss of control Failure to restrain impulses, functions, or actions that ordinarily can be regulated consciously (e.g., aggressive actions, sexual impulses, bladder and bowel emptying). In relation to alcohol and other substances, loss of control refers to an impaired ability to modulate the amount or frequency of substance intake once any amount of the substance has been administered. Such loss of control, or impaired control, is regarded as one sign of dependence on the substance used.

LSD (lysergic acid diethylamide) A potent *hallucinogen* that produces psychotic *symptoms* and behavior such as *hallucinations, illusions,* body and time-space distortions, and, less commonly, intense *panic* or mystical experiences.

lubrication-swelling response See *sexual arousal disorders.*

lumbar puncture The insertion of a needle between two of the lumbar vertebrae into the meningeal sac around the base of the spinal cord to obtain cerebrospinal fluid for diagnostic purposes.

Luria, Alexander Romanovich (1902–1977) Russian neuropsychologist who developed a treatment for *aphasia,* combining physical and psychological techniques for victims of brain trauma.

Luria-Nebraska A neuropsychological battery of tests consisting of 14 scales that assess writing, reading, arithmetic, and receptive and expressive language abilities as well as motor, tactile, auditory (rhythm), visual, memory, and intellectual functioning. The battery may detect both the presence of brain injury or abnormality and its location, and may indicate how the injury interferes with functioning.

M

magical thinking A conviction that thinking equates with doing. Occurs in dreams in children, in primitive peoples, and in patients under a variety of conditions. Characterized by lack of realistic relationship between cause and effect.

magnetic resonance imaging (MRI) A technique for showing anatomic structures that involves placing subjects in a strong magnetic field and then, by use of magnetic gradients and brief radio frequency pulses, determining the resonance characteristics at each point in the area to be studied. Used to detect structural or anatomic abnormalities; it is better able to differentiate between gray and white matter than is *computed tomography*. See *brain imaging*.

magnetoencephalography A type of *brain imaging* that measures the magnetic fields created by the electrical activity of nerve cells, both cortical and subcortical.

maintenance drug therapy Continuing a therapeutic drug after it has reached its maximum efficacy and at a minimum effective level to prevent an early relapse or a later recurrence of illness.

major affective disorders In DSM-IV called *depressive disorders* and *bipolar disorders*.

major depressive disorder See *depressive disorders*.

major epilepsy (grand mal) See under *epilepsy*.

maladjustment Unsuccessful attempts at *adaptation*.

male erectile disorder One of the *sexual arousal disorders*.

male orgasmic disorder One of the *orgasm disorders*.

maleness Anatomic and physiological features that relate to the male's procreative capacity. See *masculine*.

malingering Intentional production of false or grossly exaggerated physical or psychological *symptoms* motivated by external incentives such as avoiding onerous duties, obtaining financial compensation, evading criminal prosecution, or obtaining drugs. There is often marked discrepancy between the person's claimed disability and objective findings. The person may be uncooperative during the diagnostic evaluation or fail to comply with the prescribed treatment.

managed care A system(s) organized to create a balance between use of health care resources, control of health costs, and enhancement of the quality of care. Aiming to provide care in the most cost-effective manner, each managed care system closely monitors the intensity and duration of treatment as well as the settings in which it is provided. It adds third parties to the providers-consumers dyad to share control of the treatment process. It organizes physicians and other providers into coordinated networks of care to ensure that those who enroll in the system receive all medically necessary care. A wide array of mechanisms are used to control utilization and reduce costs.

Currently, *health maintenance organizations (HMOs)* are the most frequently used management system for managed care. In 1993, 56% of all Americans working for middle-sized and large firms were enrolled in HMOs.

mania *Bipolar disorder;* a *mood disorder* characterized by excessive elation, inflated self-esteem and *grandiosity,* hyperactivity, agitation, and accelerated thinking and speaking. *Flight of ideas* may be present. A manic syndrome may also occur in *organic mental disorders.*

–mania Formerly used as a nonspecific term for any type of "madness." Currently used as a suffix to indicate a morbid preoccupation with some kind of idea or activity, and/or a *compulsive* need to behave in some deviant way. Some examples are as follows:

egomania Pathological preoccupation with self.

erotomania The *delusion* that one is loved by a particular person.

kleptomania Compulsion to steal.

megalomania Grandiose *delusions* of power, wealth, or fame.

monomania Pathological preoccupation with one subject.

necromania Pathological preoccupation with dead bodies.

nymphomania Abnormal and excessive need or desire in the woman for sexual intercourse; see *satyriasis.*

pyromania Compulsion to set fires; an *impulse control disorder.*

trichotillomania Compulsion to pull one's own hair out; an *impulse disorder.*

maniac Imprecise, sensational, and misleading term for an emotionally disturbed person. Usually implies violent behavior. Not specifically referable to any psychiatric diagnostic category.

manic episode A distinct period of time (usually lasting at least 1 week) of abnormally and persistently elevated, expansive, or irritable mood accompanied by such *symptoms* as inflated self-esteem or *grandiosity,* decreased need for sleep, overtalkativeness or *pressured speech, flight of ideas* or feeling that thoughts are racing, inattentiveness and distractibility, increased goal-directed activity (e.g., at work or school, socially or sexually), and involvement in pleasurable activities with high potential for painful consequences (e.g., buying sprees, sexual indiscretions, foolish business ventures). See *bipolar disorders.*

manic-depressive illness A term often used synonymously with *bipolar disorder,* as defined in DSM-IV.

manifest content The remembered content of a dream or fantasy, as contrasted with *latent content,* which is concealed and distorted.

manipulation A behavior pattern characterized by attempts to exploit interpersonal contact.

MAOI See *monoamine oxidase inhibitor.*

marijuana Dried leaves and flowers of Cannabis sativa. The active intoxicating ingredient is delta-9-tetrahydrocannabinol (THC). The drug is smoked or ingested and produces *euphoria,* altered perceptions, memory impairment, and impaired *psychomotor* performance.

marital therapy A treatment whose goal is to ameliorate the problems of married couples. Various psychodynamic, sexual, ethical, and economic aspects of marriage are considered. Husband and wife are usually seen individually or conjointly. A broader term is couples therapy, which encompasses unmarried couples.

masculine A set of sex-specific social role behaviors that are unrelated to procreative biological function. See *gender identity; gender role; maleness*.

masculine protest Term coined by *Adler* to describe a striving to escape identification with the feminine role. Applies primarily to women but may also be noted in men.

masochism Pleasure derived from physical or psychological pain inflicted on oneself either by oneself or by others. It is called sexual masochism and classified as a *paraphilia* when it is consciously sought as a part of the sexual act or as a prerequisite to sexual gratification. It is the converse of *sadism*, although the two tend to coexist in the same person.

masochism, sexual One of the *paraphilias*, characterized by marked distress over, or acting on, sexual urges to be humiliated, beaten, bound, or otherwise made to suffer by the sexual partner. Among the frequently reported masochistic acts are restraint (physical bondage), blindfolding, whipping or flagellation, electrical shocks, or being treated as a helpless infant and clothed in diapers (infantilism).

maternal deprivation The result of the premature loss or absence of the mother, or the lack of proper mothering.

mathematics disorder Developmental arithmetic disorder; an *academic skills disorder* characterized by a significantly lower than expected mathematical ability given the subject's age, intelligence, and education.

maturational crises Predictable life events or turning points that occur for most individuals in the course of development.

mean See LIST OF RESEARCH TERMS.

median See LIST OF RESEARCH TERMS.

Medicaid A means-tested entitlement program, financed jointly by the state and federal governments, that provides medical services to people with low incomes. States *must* offer certain services, including inpatient and outpatient hospital services, physicians' (including psychiatrists') services, clinical laboratory and X-ray services, and home health services. Additional coverage of persons with mental illnesses is limited. For example, states *must* cover short-term acute care for mental illness in general hospitals; they *may* cover services for persons with mental illness in institutes for mental diseases for those over 65 or in psychiatric hospitals for those under 21. Institutionalized people between the ages of 21 and 65 are excluded from coverage.

medical audit See *audit.*

medical ethics The moral code adopted by health professionals in assigning primary value to their patients' needs and interests.

medical power of attorney The legal authority given by a competent person to a proxy or stand-in decision-maker to serve in the event of the subject's incapacity. This is one type of *advance directive.* See also *living will.*

medical record A written document that contains sufficient information to identify the patient clearly, to justify the diagnosis and treatment, and to document the results accurately.

medical review Examination by a team composed of physicians and other appropriate health personnel of the conditions and need for care, including a medical evaluation.

Medicare An entitlement program of health insurance for the elderly and for qualified disabled persons enacted in 1965. Part A, or hospital insurance, usually is earned through employment covered by Social Security. Part B, or supplementary medical insurance, is elected and paid for through a heavily subsidized premium. Covered services include inpatient hospital care, hospital outpatient services, skilled nursing facility care, home health care, physicians' (including psychiatrists') services, laboratory and other diagnostic tests, and hospice care.

medication-induced movement disorders See *movement disorders, medication-induced.*

megalomania See under *-mania.*

megavitamin therapy See *orthomolecular treatment.*

melancholia *Depression,* typically *endogenous* rather than reactive, and of severe degree. Some authorities use melancholia as equivalent to *depression with psychotic features.* In DSM-IV (as in DSM-III and DSM-III-R), melancholia is used as a descriptor of a major depressive episode. In addition to exhibiting loss of pleasure in activities (pervasive *anhedonia*) and lack of reaction to stimuli that would ordinarily be pleasurable, the patient often shows *psychomotor retardation* or agitation, depression that is worse in the morning, early morning awakening, *anorexia nervosa* and weight loss, and excessive or inappropriate guilt.

memory The ability, process, or act of remembering or recalling; especially the ability to reproduce what has been learned or explained.

memory consolidation The physical and psychological changes that take place as the brain organizes and restructures information that may become a permanent part of memory.

memory impairment, age-associated See *age-associated memory impairment (AAMI).*

menarche The onset of menstruation.

mendacity Pathological lying.

mental age (MA) A measure of mental ability as determined by psychological tests.

mental deficiency See *retardation, mental.*

mental disease   See *mental disorder.*

mental disorder   A behavioral or psychological *syndrome* that causes significant distress (a painful symptom) or disability (impairment in one or more important areas of functioning), or a significantly increased risk of suffering death, pain, or an important loss of freedom. The syndrome is considered to be a manifestation of some behavioral, psychological, or biological dysfunction in the person (and in some cases it is clearly secondary to or due to a *general medical condition*). The term is not applied to behavior or conflicts that arise between the person and society (e.g., politicial, religious, or sexual preference) unless such conflicts are clearly an outgrowth of a dysfunction within that person. In lay usage, "emotional illness" serves as a term for mental disorder, although it may imply a lesser degree of dysfunction, whereas the term "mental disorder" may be reserved for more severe disturbances.

mental health   A state of being that is relative rather than absolute. The best indices of mental health are simultaneous success at working, loving, and creating, with the capacity for mature and flexible resolution of conflicts between *instincts, conscience,* important other people, and reality.

mental illness   See *mental disorder.*

mental retardation   See *retardation, mental.*

mental status   The level and style of functioning of the *psyche,* including a person's intellectual functioning and emotional, attitudinal, psychological, and personality aspects and the relationships between them. The term is commonly used to refer to the results of the examination of the patient's mental state. See *association.*

mental status examination   The process of estimating psychological and behavioral function by observing the patient, eliciting his or her self-description, and using formal questioning. Included in the examination are 1) evaluation and assessment of any psychiatric condition present, including provisional *diagnosis* and *prognosis,* determination of degree of impairment, suitability for treatment, and indications for particular types of therapeutic intervention; 2) formulation of the personality structure of the subject, which may suggest the historical and developmental antecedents of whatever psychiatric condition exists; and 3) estimation of the subject's ability and willingness to participate appropriately in treatment. The mental status is reported in a series of narrative statements describing such things as *affect,* speech, thought content, perception, and *cognitive* functions. The mental status examination is part of the general examination of all patients, although it may be markedly abbreviated in the absence of *psychopathology.*

mescaline An alkaloid originally derived from the peyote cactus, resembling *amphetamine* and adrenalin chemically; used to induce altered perceptions. Also used by Native Americans of the Southwest in religious rites. See TABLE OF COMMONLY ABUSED DRUGS.

mesmerism Early term for *hypnosis.* Named after Franz Anton Mesmer (1733–1815).

mesomorphic See *constitutional types.*

metapsychiatry The interface between *psychiatry* and such psychic phenomena as *parapsychology,* mysticism, altered states of consciousness, and nonmedical healing.

metapsychology The branch of theoretical or speculative *psychology* that deals with the significance of mental processes; the nature of the mind-body relationship; the origin, purpose, and structure of the mind; and similar hypotheses that are beyond the realm of empirical verification.

methadone A synthetic *narcotic.* It may be used as a substitute for heroin, producing a less socially disabling *addiction* or aiding in the withdrawal from heroin. It may be abused. See *narcotic-blocking drugs* and TABLE OF COMMONLY ABUSED DRUGS.

Meyer, Adolf (1866–1950) Swiss-born American *psychiatrist,* professor of psychiatry at Johns Hopkins University; introduced the concept of *psychobiology.* See OUTLINE OF SCHOOLS OF PSYCHIATRY.

MHPG (3-methoxy-4-hydroxyphenylglycol) A major metabolite of brain *norepinephrine* excreted in urine.

middle age Conventionally considered to occur between 40 and 60–65 years of age and primarily defined by *psychosocial* rather than by physiological events.

midlife crisis The set of problems that arise when individuals discover visible signs that they are aging and become preoccupied with the realization.

migraine A *syndrome* characterized by recurrent, severe, and usually one-sided headaches; often associated with nausea, vomiting, and visual disturbances.

milieu therapy Socioenvironmental therapy in which the attitudes and behavior of the staff of a treatment service and the activities prescribed for the patients are determined by the patients' emotional and interpersonal needs. This therapy is an essential part of all inpatient treatment.

minimal brain dysfunction (MBD) An older term, currently out of favor, for *attention-deficit/hyperactivity disorder (ADHD).* It begins in childhood and persists into adolescence, and sometimes into adulthood. Characterized by decreased attention span, distractibility, increased activity, impulsivity, emotional *lability,* poor motor integration, disturbances in perception, and disorders of language development. See *learning disability.*

Minnesota Multiphasic Personality Inventory (MMPI) See TABLE OF PSYCHOLOGICAL TESTS.

minor depressive disorder See *depressive disorders.*

minor epilepsy (petit mal) See under *epilepsy.*

mirroring 1) The empathic responsiveness of the parent to the developing child's grandiose-exhibitionistic needs. Parental expressions of delight in the child's activities signal that the child's wishes and experiences are accepted as legitimate. This teaches the child which of his or her potential qualities are most highly esteemed and valued. Mirroring validates the child as to who he or she is and affirms his or her worth. The process transforms archaic aims to realizable aims, and it determines in part the content of the self-assessing, self-monitoring functions and their relationships to the rest of the *personality.* The content of the *superego* is the residue of the mirroring experience. See *grandiose self.* 2) A technique in *psychodrama* in which another person in the group plays the role of the patient, who watches the enactment as if gazing into a mirror. The first person may exaggerate one or more aspects of the patient's behavior. Following the portrayal, the patient is usually encouraged to comment on what he or she has observed.

Mitchell, S. Weir (1829–1914) American *neurologist* who described *causalgia* and developed a once popular "rest cure" for patients with emotional disorders.

mixed anxiety-depressive disorder Symptoms of *anxiety* and *depression* that cause significant impairment or distress but do not meet the criteria for an *anxiety disorder* or a *mood disorder.*

mixed receptive/expressive language disorder See *communication disorders.*

M'Naughten rule See under *insanity defense* in LIST OF LEGAL TERMS.

mode See LIST OF RESEARCH TERMS.

modeling Learning by imitation; a form of *behavior therapy* based on social learning in which the model (e.g., the therapist, an actor, or someone else the patient views as competent) displays the desired behavior, the patient repeats it, and successful repetitions are reinforced.

molecular biology The level of biology concerned with the study of structures and processes at the cellular level, and particularly of intracellular responses such as the role of a protein, enzyme, and other chemicals in a metabolic pathway, how nucleic acid stores information affecting cellular structure and function, and how metabolites in one cell may affect the function of other cells.

mongolism See *Down syndrome.*

monoamine An *amine* containing only one amino group.

monoamine oxidase (MAO) A brain or liver enzyme that breaks down *biogenic amines* (*neurotransmitters*), rendering them inactive. Inhibition of this enzyme by certain antidepressant drugs (*monoamine oxidase inhibitor*s) may result in alleviation of depressed states. See *biogenic amines* and TABLE OF DRUGS USED IN PSYCHIATRY.

monoamine oxidase inhibitor (MAOI) A group of antidepressant drugs that inhibit the enzyme *monoamine oxidase (MAO)* in the brain and raise the levels of *biogenic amines*. See TABLE OF DRUGS USED IN PSYCHIATRY.

monomania See under -*mania.*

monozygotic twins Twins who develop from a single fertilized ovum; identical twins. Often referred to as MZ twins, in contrast to DZ twins (*dizygotic twins*).

mood See *affect.*

mood disorder due to a general medical condition Secondary mood disorder; prominent and persistent *depression* (with depressed mood or loss of interest or pleasure) or *mania* (elevated, expansive, or irritable mood), or both, associated with a medical condition classified outside the ICD-10 list of mental disorders.

mood disorders In DSM-IV, this category includes *depressive disorders, bipolar disorders, mood disorder due to a general medical condition,* and substance-induced (intoxication/withdrawal) mood disorder.

mood swing Fluctuation of a person's emotional tone between periods of elation and periods of depression.

mood-congruent psychotic features See *depression with psychotic features; manic episode.*

mood-incongruent psychotic features See *depression with psychotic features; manic episode.*

moral treatment A philosophy and technique of treating mental patients that began to prevail in the first half of the 19th century and emphasized removal of restraints, humane and kindly care, attention to religion, and performance by the patients of useful tasks in the hospital.

motor skills disorder Includes developmental coordination disorder, which is characterized by poor performance in activities requiring motor coordination. Performance is below that expected given the subject's age and intelligence. Examples are delays in achieving motor milestones such as walking, crawling, or sitting; clumsiness; lack of expected proficiency in sports; or poor handwriting.

motor tic disorder See *tic disorders.*

mourning *Grief;* reaction to a loss of a love object (i.e., important person, object, role, status, or anything considered part of one's life) consisting of a process of emotional detachment from that object which frees the subject to find other interests and enjoyments.

movement disorders, medication-induced In DSM-IV, this group includes *neuroleptic malignant syndrome, parkinsonism, akathisia, tardive dyskinesia, dystonia,* and *tremor.*

MPD *Multiple personality disorder.* See *dissociative disorders.*

MRI See *magnetic resonance imaging.*

multi-infarct dementia See *dementia, vascular*.

multiple personality disorder In DSM-IV, this has been renamed dissociative identity disorder (multiple personality disorder). It consists of the existence within one person of two or more distinct personalities or personality states (alters or alter personalities). Each personality state has its own relatively enduring pattern of perceiving, relating to, and thinking about the environment and the self, and at least two of them alternate in taking control of the person's behavior. Characteristically, there is an amnesic barrier between personalities, which may be absolute or, more commonly, unilateral, denying one personality access to the memories of the other, but allowing the other personality full access to the memory systems of both.

Munchausen syndrome (pathomimicry) In DSM-IV, a chronic form of *factitious disorder* with physical symptoms that may be totally fabricated, self-inflicted, or exaggerations of preexisting physical conditions. The subject's entire life may consist of seeking admission to or staying in hospitals (often under different names). Multiple invasive procedures and operations are eagerly solicited. The need is to assume the sick role, rather than to reap any economic benefit or ensure better care or physical well-being.

mutation A change in genetic structure that produces transmissible, permanent differences. May occur spontaneously or may be induced by such agents as high-energy radiation. See *genes*.

mutism Refusal to speak; may be for *conscious* or *unconscious* reasons.

mutism, selective Elective mutism; a disorder of infancy, childhood, or adolescence characterized by persistent failure to speak in specific social situations by a child with demonstrated ability to speak. The mutism is not due to lack of fluency in the language being spoken or embarrassment about a speech problem.

mysophobia See *phobia*.

N

naloxone A potent but short-acting narcotic *antagonist* with no *agonistic* effects of its own; the drug of choice in the treatment of narcotic overdose. Its short duration of action (2 to 4 hours) makes it generally inappropriate for chronic treatment of narcotic *addiction*.

naltrexone A long-acting opiate-blocking drug usually given orally. The effects of opiates, including euphoria, are blocked, which may lead to the extinction of continued drug-seeking behaviors.

narcissism Self-love as opposed to object-love (love of another person). In classical psychoanalytic theory (see *psychoanalysis*), *cathexis* (investment) of the psychic representation of the self with *libido* (sexual interest and energy). An excess of narcissism interferes with relations with others. To be distinguished from egotism, which carries the connotation of self-centeredness, selfishness, and conceit. Egotism is but one expression of narcissism. Recent revisions in psychoanalytic theory (*self psychology*) have viewed the concept of narcissism in less pathological terms.

narcissistic personality disorder See *personality disorder*.

narcissistic rage Reactive aggression in a person with a defective self structure, provoked by injuries to the self such as deflation of infantile grandiosity or traumatic disappointment in idealized figures. The aggression may range from mild annoyance to intense and violent destruction. See *fragmentation; grandiose self; idealized parental imago.*

narcoanalysis See *narcosynthesis.*

narcolepsy A *dyssomnia* consisting of irresistible attacks of refreshing *sleep* during the day, *cataplexy* (sudden bilateral loss of muscle tone) typically associated with intense emotion, and recurrent intrusions of REM sleep into the transition between sleep and wakefulness.

narcosis Stupor of varying depth induced by certain drugs.

narcosynthesis Psychotherapeutic treatment under partial *anesthesia,* such as that induced by *barbiturates.* Originally used to treat acute *mental disorders* occurring in a military combat setting.

narcotic Any opiate derivative drug, natural or synthetic, that relieves pain or alters *mood.* May cause *addiction.* See also *drug dependence; hypnotic; sedative.*

narcotic-blocking drugs (narcotic antagonists) Agents structurally similar to the opiates and probably occupying the same receptor sites in the *central nervous system.* In sufficient doses they block the effects of opiate drugs by competing for receptor sites. If given after opiate dependence has developed, they will precipitate an acute *abstinence* syndrome. See *naloxone; naltrexone.*

National Alliance for the Mentally Ill (NAMI) An organization whose members are parents and relatives of mentally ill patients and former patients whose main objective is for better and more sustained care. Its trustees and chapter officers engage in active lobbying and in education projects.

National Institutes of Health An agency of the U.S. Department of Health and Human Services that is a world-renowned institution supporting biomedical and behavioral research. Its components are the National Cancer Institute; the National Heart, Lung, and Blood Institute; the National Library of Medicine; the National Institute of Diabetes and Digestive and Kidney Diseases; the National Institute of Allergy and Infectious Diseases; the National Institute of Child Health and Human Development; the National Institute on Deafness and Other Communication Disorders; the National Institute of Dental Research; the National Institute of Environmental Health Sciences; the National Institute of General Medical Sciences; the National Institute of Neurological Disorders and Stroke; the National Eye Institute; the National Institute on Aging; the National Institute of Arthritis and Musculoskeletal and Skin Diseases; the Clinical Center; the Fogarty International Center; the National Center for Human Genome Research; the National Center for Nursing Research; the Division of Computer Research and Technology; the National Center for Research Resources; and the Division of Research Grants. In 1992, the *National Institute of Mental Health,* the National Institute on Drug Abuse, and the National Institute on Alcoholism and Alcohol Abuse were added.

National Institute of Mental Health (NIMH) An institute within the *National Institutes of Health* responsible for research on the causes and treatments of mental illnesses.

National Mental Health Association (NMHA) Leading voluntary citizens' organization in the mental health field; formerly called the National Association for Mental Health; founded in 1909 by Clifford W. *Beers* as the National Committee for Mental Hygiene.

necromania See under *-mania.*

necrophilia One of the *paraphilias,* characterized by marked distress over, or acting on, urges involving sexual activity with corpses.

negative symptoms Most commonly refers to a group of symptoms characteristic of *schizophrenia* that include loss of fluency and spontaneity of verbal expression, impaired ability to focus or sustain attention on a particular task, difficulty in initiating or following through on tasks, impaired ability to experience pleasure to form emotional attachment to others, and blunted *affect*.

negative therapeutic reaction Obstinate resistance to change in psychoanalytic therapy. The patient's *neurotic* behavior increases after an improvement in therapy, and he or she gets worse instead of improving as would be expected. The patient seems to prefer suffering to being cured. Because such a reaction seemed to defy the *pleasure principle, Freud* related the reaction to *unconscious* guilt and *masochism,* and to the workings of the *death instinct.*

negativism Opposition or resistance, either covert or overt, to outside suggestions or advice. May be seen in *schizophrenia.*

negativistic personality disorder A type of *passive-aggressive personality disorder* characterized by passive resistance to demands for adequate social and occupational performance and a negative attitude. Typical manifestations include inefficiency, procrastination, complaints of being victimized and unappreciated, irritability, criticism of and scorn for authority, and personal discontent. The person with this disorder alternates between hostile assertions of independence and contrite, dependent behavior.

neologism In *psychiatry,* a new word or condensed combination of several words coined by a person to express a highly complex idea not readily understood by others; seen in *schizophrenia* and *organic mental disorders.*

nervous breakdown A nonmedical, nonspecific euphemism for a *mental disorder.*

neurasthenia One of the *somatoform disorders,* characterized by persisting complaints of mental or physical fatigue or weakness after performing daily activities and inability to recover with normal periods of rest or entertainment. Typical *symptoms* include muscular aches and pains, dizziness, tension headaches, sleep disturbance, and irritability.

neurochemistry The branch of chemistry that deals with the nervous system, including its chemical components and the passage of the nerve impulse through the nerve cell and its transmission across synapses.

neuroendocrinology The science of the relationships between the nervous system (particularly the brain) and the endocrine system. Of particular importance is the action of the *hypothalamus,* which stimulates or inhibits the pituitary secretion of hormones.

neurohormone A chemical messenger usually produced within the *hypothalamus,* carried to the pituitary, and then to other cells within the *central nervous system.* Neurohormones are similar to *neurotransmitters* except that they interact with a variety of cells, whereas neurotransmitters interact only with other *neurons.*

neuroleptic An antipsychotic drug. See also TABLE OF DRUGS USED IN PSYCHIATRY.

neuroleptic malignant syndrome A severe medication-induced *movement disorder* associated with the use of a neuroleptic medication. *Symptoms* include muscle rigidity, high fever, and related findings such as *dysphagia,* incontinence, confusion, or *mutism.*

neurologic disorders See LIST OF NEUROLOGIC DEFICITS.

neurologist A physician with postgraduate training and experience in the field of organic diseases of the nervous system whose professional work focuses primarily on this area. Neurologists also receive training in *psychiatry.*

neurology The branch of medical science devoted to the study, diagnosis, and treatment of organic diseases of the nervous system.

neuron A nerve cell.

neurophysiology The study of the relationship between the structure of the nervous system and its function.

neuropsychiatry The medical specialty that combines *neurology* and *psychiatry*, emphasizing the somatic substructure on which emotions are based and the organic disturbances of the *central nervous system* that give rise to *mental disorders*.

neuroreceptors Binding sites in the *central nervous system* for psychoactive drugs, *neurotransmitters*, and hormones.

neuroscience The study of brain function and the neural substrates of behavior. This interdisciplinary field includes investigation in areas such as anatomy, *genetics, biochemistry, psychiatry*, and computer science.

neurosis In common usage, emotional disturbances of all kinds other than *psychosis*. It implies subjective psychological pain or discomfort beyond what is appropriate in the conditions of one's life. The meaning of the term has been changed since it was first introduced into standard nomenclature. As currently used, some clinicians limit the term to its descriptive meaning, *neurotic disorder*, whereas others include the concept of a specific etiological process (see *etiology*). Common neuroses are as follows:

    anxiety neurosis Chronic and persistent apprehension manifested by autonomic hyperactivity (sweating, palpitations, dizziness, etc.), musculoskeletal tension, and irritability. Somatic symptoms may be prominent.

    depersonalization neurosis Feelings of unreality and of estrangement from the self, body, or surroundings. Different from the process of *deperson-alization,* which may be a manifestation of *anxiety* or of another *mental disorder.*

depressive neurosis An outmoded term for excessive reaction of *depression* due to an internal *conflict* or to an identifiable event such as loss of a loved one or of a cherished possession.

hysterical neurosis, conversion type Disorders of the special senses or the voluntary nervous system, such as blindness, deafness, *anesthesia, paresthesia,* pain, paralysis, and impaired muscle coordination. A patient with this disorder may show *la belle indifférence* to the symptoms, which may actually provide *secondary gains* by winning the patient sympathy or relief from unpleasant responsibilities. See also *conversion.*

hysterical neurosis, dissociative type Alterations in the state of consciousness or in identity, producing such symptoms as *amnesia.*

obsessive-compulsive neurosis Persistent intrusion of unwanted and uncontrollable *ego-dystonic* thoughts, urges, or actions. The thoughts may consist of single words, ruminations, or trains of thought that are seen as nonsensical. The actions may vary from simple movements to complex rituals, such as repeated handwashing. See also *compulsion.*

phobic neurosis An intense fear of an object or situation that the person consciously recognizes as harmless. Apprehension may be experienced as faintness, fatigue, palpitations, perspiration, nausea, tremor, and even *panic.* See also *phobia.*

neurotic disorder A *mental disorder* in which the predominant disturbance is a distressing *symptom* or group of symptoms that one considers unacceptable and alien to one's personality. There is no marked loss of *reality testing;* behavior does not actively violate gross social norms, although it may be quite disabling. The disturbance is relatively enduring or recurrent without treatment and is not limited to a mild transitory reaction to *stress*. There is no demonstrable organic *etiology*. See also *neurotic process*.

neurotic process A specific etiological process involving the following sequence: *unconscious conflicts* between opposing wishes or between wishes and prohibitions lead to unconscious perception of anticipated danger or *dysphoria,* which leads to use of *defense mechanisms* that result in either *symptoms, personality* disturbance, or both. See also *neurosis; neurotic disorder.*

neurotoxin A substance that is poisonous or destructive to nerve tissue.

neurotransmitter A chemical (e.g., *acetylcholine, GABA, dopamine, norepinephrine, serotonin)* found in the nervous system that facilitates the transmission of impulses across *synapses* between *neurons.* Disorders in the brain physiology of neurotransmitters have been implicated in the actions of drugs used to treat several psychiatric illnesses, particularly *mood disorders* and *schizophrenia.*

nicotine use disorders In DSM-IV this group includes nicotine dependence and nicotine withdrawal.

night hospital See *partial hospitalization.*

night terror (pavor nocturnus) See *sleep terror disorder.*

nightmare disorder Dream anxiety disorder; a *parasomnia* consisting of repeated awakenings from *sleep* with detailed recall of extended and extremely frightening dreams, usually involving threats to survival, security, or self-esteem. Upon awakening from the frightening dream, the person rapidly becomes oriented and alert. This contrasts with the confusion and disorientation characteristic of *sleep terror disorder* and some forms of *epilepsy*. Nightmares generally occur during the second half of the sleep period.

nihilistic delusion The *delusion* of nonexistence of the self or part of the self, or of some object in external reality.

nitrites "Poppers" or nitrite inhalants, including amyl, butyl, and isobutyl nitrite, that produce an intoxication characterized by a feeling of fullness in the head, mild *euphoria,* a change in the perception of time, relaxation of smooth muscles, and possibly an increase in sexual feelings. The nitrites may produce psychological dependence and may impair immune functioning, irritate the respiratory system, and induce a toxic reaction involving vomiting, severe headache, and dizziness.

nitrous oxide Laughing gas; it rapidly produces intoxication, with light-headedness and a floating sensation. *Symptoms* disappear within minutes after discontinuation of the substance, but regular use has been followed by temporary but clinically relevant confusion and reversible *paranoid* states.

nocturnal myoclonus See *dyssomnias.*

norepinephrine A *catecholamine neurotransmitter* related to *epinephrine.* It is found in both the peripheral nervous system and the *central nervous system.* Functional excesses in the brain have been implicated in the pathogenesis of manic states (see *mania*); functional deficits, in certain depressive states. Also called noradrenaline. See also *biogenic amines.*

nosology Science of the classification of disorders.

NREM sleep Non-REM sleep. See *sleep.*

nuclear family Immediate members of a family.

nuclear magnetic resonance (NMR) See *magnetic resonance imaging* (MRI); see also *brain imaging.*

nuclear self See *bipolar self.*

null hypothesis The assumption that any difference found between two samples or populations is due to chance rather than to a systematic variation. See LIST OF RESEARCH TERMS.

nursing care plan A means of providing nursing personnel with information about the needs of and therapeutic strategy for each patient.

nymphomania See under *-mania.*

nystagmus Abnormal movements of the eyeballs; side to side (horizontal), up and down (vertical), or circularly (rotary). Such movements suggest organic pathology of the *central nervous system* or of the oculomotor, trochlear, or abducens cranial nerves. Seen in toxic states such as intoxication with alcohol, sedative/hypnotic/anxiolytic drugs, inhalants, or phencyclidine.

O

object relations The emotional bonds between one person and another, as contrasted with interest in and love for the self; usually described in terms of capacity for loving and reacting appropriately to others. Melanie *Klein* is generally credited with founding the British object-relations school.

obsession Recurrent and persistent thought, impulse, or image experienced as intrusive and distressing. Recognized as being excessive and unreasonable even though it is the product of one's mind. This thought, impulse, or image cannot be expunged by logic or reasoning.

obsessive-compulsive disorder An *anxiety disorder* characterized by obsessions, compulsions, or both, that are time-consuming and interfere significantly with normal routine, occupational functioning, usual social activities, or relationships with others. See *compulsion; obsession.*

obsessive-compulsive neurosis See *neurosis*.

obsessive-compulsive personality disorder See *personality disorder*.

occupational problem Job or work difficulty that is not due to a *mental disorder*. Examples are job dissatisfaction or uncertainty about career choices.

occupational psychiatry (industrial psychiatry) A field of *psychiatry* concerned with the diagnosis and prevention of *mental illness* in industry, with the return of the psychiatric patient to work, and with psychiatric aspects of absenteeism, abuse, retirement, and related phenomena. A psychiatrist in this field often works in consultation to an *employee assistance program (EAP)*.

occupational therapy An adjunctive therapy that utilizes purposeful activities as a means of altering the course of illness. The patient's relationship to staff and to other patients in the occupational therapy setting is often more therapeutic than the activity itself.

Oedipus complex Attachment of the child to the parent of the opposite sex, accompanied by envious and aggressive feelings toward the parent of the same sex. These feelings are largely repressed (i.e., made *unconscious*) because of the fear of displeasure or punishment by the parent of the same sex. In its original use, the term applied only to the boy or man.

onanism Coitus interruptus. The term is sometimes used interchangeably with masturbation.

ontogenetic Pertaining to the development of the individual. Contrast with *phylogenetic*.

operant conditioning (instrumental conditioning) A process by which the results of the person's behavior determine whether the behavior is more or less likely to occur in the future. See also *respondent conditioning; shaping*.

opiate Any chemical derived from opium; relieves pain and produces a sense of well-being.

opioid A drug or naturally occurring substance that resembles opium or one or more of its alkaloid derivatives.

opioid use disorders In DSM-IV, this group includes opioid dependence, opioid abuse, opioid intoxication, opioid withdrawal, opioid delirium, opioid psychotic disorder with delusions or hallucinations, opioid mood disorder, opioid sexual dysfunction, and opioid sleep disorder.

oppositional defiant disorder A pattern of negativistic and hostile behavior in a child that lasts at least 6 months. *Symptoms* may include losing one's temper; arguing with adults or actively refusing their requests; deliberately annoying others; being easily annoyed, angry, and resentful; and being spiteful or vindictive.

oral phase See *psychosexual development.*

organic brain syndrome See *organic mental disorder.*

organic disease A disease characterized by demonstrable structural or biochemical abnormality in an organ or tissue. Sometimes imprecisely used as an antonym for *functional disorder.*

organic mental disorder A condition showing behavioral or psychological *symptoms* that is secondary to or based upon detectable disturbances in brain tissue functioning. Recent advances in *genetics, neurophysiology,* and *brain imaging* make possible identifying a number of biological and physiological factors that contribute to many traditionally "nonorganic" mental disorders. Consequently, there is general agreement that it is difficult, if not impossible, to make clear distinctions between "organic" and "nonorganic." DSM-IV includes *delirium, dementia,* and *amnestic disorders* in a section labeled "Cognitive Disorders." The remaining disorders in DSM-III-R labeled "organic" (mood, anxiety, personality, and delusional disorders, and "organic" hallucinosis) are placed in

DSM-IV within the diagnostic categories with which they share phenomenology and are identified as substance-induced or due to a *general medical condition.*

orgasm Sexual climax; peak psychophysiological response to sexual stimulation.

orgasm disorders One group of *sexual dysfunctions* including female orgasmic disorder, male orgasmic disorder, and premature ejaculation.

female orgasmic disorder (inhibited female orgasm) Refers to absence of, or delay in attaining, orgasm following a normal sexual excitement phase. The orgasmic capacity is less than would be expected for the woman's age, sexual experience, and the degree or type of sexual stimulation. It is frequently severe enough to cause marked distress or interpersonal difficulty. The disorder is termed "generalized" if it is present in all situations and "situational" if the woman is orgasmic under some conditions or with some partners.

male orgasmic disorder (inhibited male orgasm) Refers to absence of, or delay in attaining, orgasm following a normal sexual excitement phase during sexual activity that is adequate in focus, intensity, and duration. In the older literature, absence of orgasm was often termed *ejaculatory incompetence (impotence),* and delayed orgasm was called ejaculatio retardata.

premature ejaculation Refers to ejaculation following minimal sexual stimulation before, at the point of, or shortly after entry and before the man wishes it.

orgasmic dysfunction Inability of the woman to achieve *orgasm* through physical stimulation. Masters and Johnson described two types of orgasmic dysfunction. In primary orgasmic dysfunction, the woman has never had an orgasm through any physical contact, including masturbation. In situational orgasmic dysfunction, there has been at least one instance of orgasm through physical contact. Compare with *impotence.*

orientation   Awareness of one's self in relation to time, place, and person.

orphan drugs   Drugs that the pharmaceutical companies do not wish to develop either because they cannot be patented (e.g., lithium), because they are used only in rare conditions by very few people, or because of a variety of legitimate economic reasons. In such cases, the federal government will work with the companies to make the drugs available to those persons who need them.

orthomolecular treatment (megavitamin therapy)   An approach based on the assumption that "for every twisted mind there is a twisted molecule" and that in some way psychiatric illness, and perhaps other illnesses, are due to biochemical abnormalities, resulting in increased needs for specific substances, such as vitamins. This treatment is of unknown and unproved efficacy.

orthopsychiatry   An approach that involves the collaborative efforts of *psychiatry, psychology, psychiatric social work,* and other behavioral, medical, and social sciences in the study and treatment of human behavior in the clinical setting. Emphasis is placed on preventive techniques to promote healthy emotional growth and development, particularly of children.

outpatient   A patient who is receiving ambulatory care at a hospital or other health facility without being admitted to the facility.

overanxious disorder   An anxiety disorder of childhood and adolescence, sometimes considered equivalent to the adult diagnosis of *generalized anxiety disorder. Symptoms* include multiple, unrealistic anxieties concerning the quality of one's performance in school and in sports; hobbies; money matters; punctuality; health; or appearance. The patient is tense and unable to relax and has recurrent somatic complaints for which no physical cause can be found.

overcompensation A *conscious* or *unconscious* process in which a real or imagined physical or psychological deficit generates exaggerated correction. Concept introduced by *Adler.*

overdetermination The concept of multiple *unconscious* causes of an emotional reaction or *symptom.*

overstimulation Excitation that exceeds the subject's or the system's ability to master it or to discharge it. In accordance with the *economic viewpoint,* the psyche has a finite capacity for tension. When that capacity is exceeded, the psyche feels pain (*anxiety*) and the excessive stimulation constitutes a trauma. Eventually, anxiety becomes a signal that danger is approaching, and defenses against being overwhelmed are brought forth (see *signal anxiety*). The adult is able to master more stimulation than the child, but even the mature psyche cannot cope with an unlimited amount of increasing or repeated overstimulation.

P

pain disorder One of the *somatoform disorders,* characterized by pain in one or more sites that causes marked distress or impairs occupational or social functioning. The pain may occur in the absence of any physical finding that might explain it (psychological type), or it may be related to an existing *general medical condition.*

pandemic See under *epidemiology.*

panic Sudden, overwhelming *anxiety* of such intensity that it produces terror and physiological changes.

panic attack A period of intense fear or discomfort, with the abrupt development of a variety of *symptoms* and fears of dying, going crazy, or losing control that reach a crescendo within 10 minutes. The symptoms may include shortness of breath or smothering sensations; dizziness, faintness, or feelings of unsteadiness; trembling or shaking; sweating; choking; nausea or abdominal distress; flushes or chills; and chest pain or discomfort.

Panic attacks occur in several *anxiety disorders*. In *panic disorder* they are typically unexpected and happen "out of the blue." In *social phobia* and *simple phobia* they are cued and occur when exposed to or in anticipation of a situational trigger. These attacks occur also in *posttraumatic stress disorder*.

panic disorder Recurrent, unexpected *panic attacks,* at least one of which is followed by a month or more of persisting concern about having these attacks. There are two types of panic disorder: with or without *agoraphobia*.

panphobia See *phobia*.

paranoia A condition characterized by the gradual development of an intricate, complex, and elaborate system of thinking based on (and often proceeding logically from) misinterpretation of an actual event; a *delusional disorder*. Despite its chronic course, this condition does not seem to interfere with thinking and personality. To be distinguished from *schizophrenia, paranoid type*.

paranoid A lay term commonly used to describe an overly suspicious person. The technical use of the term refers to persons with *paranoid ideation* or to a type of *schizophrenia* or a class of disorders. See also *delusional disorder*.

paranoid disorders See *delusional disorder*.

paranoid ideation Suspiciousness or nondelusional belief that one is being harassed, persecuted, or unfairly treated.

paranoid personality disorder See *personality disorder.*

paranoid schizophrenia See *schizophrenia.*

paraphilias One of the major groups of *sexual disorders;* in DSM-IV, this group includes *exhibitionism, fetishism, frotteurism, pedophilia, sexual masochism,* sexual sadism, voyeurism, *transvestic fetishism,* and paraphilia not otherwise specified, which includes *necrophilia* and *klismaphilia.*

The paraphilias (also called *perversions* or sexual deviations) are recurrent, intense sexual urges and sexually arousing fantasies that involve nonhuman objects, children or other nonconsenting persons, or the suffering or humiliation of oneself or the sexual partner.

parapraxis A faulty act, blunder, or lapse of memory such as a slip of the tongue or misplacement of an article. According to *Freud,* these acts are caused by *unconscious* motives.

paraprofessional A trained aide who assists a professional person, usually in a medical setting.

parapsychology The study of sensory and motor phenomena shown by some human beings (and some animals) that occur without the mediation of the known sensory and motor organs. The data of parapsychology are not accounted for by the tenets of conventional science. See *extrasensory perception; telepathy.*

parasomnias One group of *sleep disorders;* in DSM-IV, this group includes *nightmare disorder, sleep terror disorder,* and *sleepwalking disorder.* The other group of sleep disorders is *dyssomnias.*

parasympathetic nervous system The part of the *autonomic nervous system* that controls the life-sustaining organs of the body under normal, danger-free conditions and is mediated by *acetylcholine*. See also *sympathetic nervous system.*

parataxic distortion *Sullivan's* term for inaccuracies in *judgment* and *perception,* particularly in inter-personal relations, based on the observer's need to perceive subjects and relationships in accordance with a pattern set by earlier experience. Parataxic distortions develop as a *defense* against *anxiety.*

parent-child relational problem See *relational problems.*

paresis Weakness of organic origin; incomplete paralysis; term often used instead of *general paralysis.*

paresthesia Abnormal tactile sensation, often described as burning, pricking, tickling, tingling, or creeping.

parkinsonism (Parkinson's disease, paralysis agitans) One of the *medication-induced movement disorders,* consisting of a rapid, coarse tremor; muscular ridigity; or *akinesia* developing within a few weeks of starting or raising the dose of neuroleptic medication, or of reducing medication used to treat *extrapyramidal symptoms.*

partial hospitalization A psychiatric treatment program for patients who require hospitalization only during the day, overnight, or on weekends.

partner relational problem See *relational problems.*

passive-aggressive personality See *personality disorder.*

passive-dependent personality See *dependent* personality under *personality disorder.*

pastoral counseling The use of psychological principles by clergy trained to assist members of their congregation who seek help with emotional problems.

pathognomonic A *symptom* or group of symptoms that are specifically diagnostic or typical of a disease.

Pavlov, Ivan Petrovich (1849–1936) Russian neuro-physiologist noted for his research on *conditioning*. He was awarded the Nobel Prize in Medicine (1904) for his work on the physiology of digestion.

pavor nocturnus See *sleep terror disorder*.

PCP *Phencyclidine*.

PDD Primary degenerative dementia. See *Alzheimer's disease*.

pederasty *Homosexual* anal intercourse between men and boys with the latter as the passive partners. The term is used less precisely to denote male homosexual anal intercourse.

pedophilia One of the *paraphilias,* characterized by marked distress over, or acting on, urges involving sexual activity with a prepubescent child who, more often than not, is of the same sex.

peeping See *voyeurism*.

peer review Review by panels of physicians, and sometimes allied health professionals, of services rendered by other physicians. See also *professional standards review organization; utilization review committee*.

peer review organization (PRO) A system that determines the appropriateness and reasonableness of medical care under the Medicare program.

pellagra A vitamin B$_3$ (nicotinamide) deficiency that may be a cause of major mental *symptoms* such as *delusions* and impaired thinking, as well as physical symptoms such as dermatitis.

penis envy In psychoanalytic theory (see *psychoanalysis*), envy by the female child of the male child's genitals and the presumably associated powers or privileges.

perception Mental processes by which intellectual, sensory, and emotional data are organized logically or meaningfully.

periaqueductal gray area A cluster of neurons lying in the thalamus and pons. It contains endorphin-producing *neurons* and opiate receptor sites and thus can affect the sensation of pain.

persecutory delusion See *delusional disorder*.

perseveration See LIST OF NEUROLOGIC DEFICITS.

persona A Jungian term for the personality mask or facade that each person presents to the outside world, as distinguished from the person's inner being, or *anima* (animus). See *Jung*.

personality The characteristic way in which a person thinks, feels, and behaves; the ingrained pattern of behavior that each person evolves, both consciously and unconsciously, as his or her style of life or way of being.

personality change disorders Alterations in characteristic patterns of relating to the environment and the self that occur from social, psychological, or physical stressors such as having catastrophic experiences, having a *mental disorder,* or having a *general medical condition* (e.g., brain trauma). The personality shows a definite change from the preexisting personality; in children, there is a significant change from usual behavior patterns or a disruption in development. Features appear that were not present earlier such as a hostile, mistrustful, or suspicious attitude; social withdrawal; feelings of emptiness or hopelessness; or poor impulse control or aggressive behavior.

personality disorder Enduring patterns of perceiving, relating to, and thinking about the environment and oneself that begin by early adulthood and are exhibited in a wide range of important social and personal contexts. These patterns are inflexible and maladaptive, causing either significant functional impairment or subjective distress.

Many types of personality or personality disorder have been described. The following include those specified in DSM-IV, which groups them into three clusters:

Cluster A paranoid, schizoid, schizotypal

Cluster B antisocial, borderline, histrionic, narcissistic

Cluster C avoidant, dependent, obsessive-compulsive

antisocial In the older literature called *psychopathic personality,* descriptions have tended to emphasize either antisocial behavior or interpersonal and affectional inadequacies, each at the expense of the other. Among the more commonly cited descriptors are superficiality; lack of empathy and remorse, with callous unconcern for the feelings of others; disregard for social norms; poor behavioral controls, with irritability, impulsivity, and low frustration tolerance; and inability to feel guilt or to learn from experience or punishment. Often, there is evidence of conduct disorder (*disruptive behavior disorder*) in childhood or of overtly irresponsible and antisocial behavior in adulthood, such as inability to sustain consistent work behavior, conflicts with the law, repeated failure to meet financial obligations, and repeated lying or "conning" of others.

avoidant Characterized by social discomfort and reticence, low self-esteem, and hypersensitivity to negative evaluation. Manifestations may include avoiding activities that involve contact with others because of fears of criticism or disapproval; experiencing inhibited development of relationships with others because of fears of being foolish or being shamed; having few friends despite the desire to relate to others; or being unusually reluctant to take personal risks or engage in new activities because they may prove embarrassing.

borderline Characterized by instability of interpersonal relationships, self-image, *affects,* and control over impulses. Manifestations may include frantic efforts to avoid real or imagined abandonment; unstable, intense relationships that alternate between extremes of *idealization* and *devaluation;* recurrent self-mutilation or *suicide* threats; and inappropriate, intense, or uncontrolled anger.

dependent Characterized by an excessive need to be taken care of, resulting in submissive and clinging behavior and fears of separation. Manifestations may include excessive need for advice and reassurances about everyday decisions, encouragement of others to assume responsibility for major areas of his or her life, inability to express disagreement because of possible anger or lack of support from others, and preoccupation with fears of being left to take care of himself or herself.

histrionic Characterized by excessive emotional instability and attention seeking. Behavior includes discomfort if not the center of attention; overattention to physical attractiveness; rapidly shifting and shallow emotions; speech that is excessively impressionistic and lacking in detail; viewing relationships as being more intimate than they actually are; and seeking immediate gratification.

narcissistic Characterized by a pervasive pattern of *grandiosity* in fantasy or behavior and an excessive need for admiration. Manifestations may include having an exaggerated sense of self-importance, having a feeling of being special so that he or she should associate only with other special people, exploiting others to advance his or her own ends, lacking *empathy,* and often believing that others envy him or her.

obsessive-compulsive Also compulsive personality; characterized by preoccupation with perfectionism, mental and interpersonal control, and orderliness, all at the expense of flexibility, openness, and efficiency. Some of the manifestations are preoccupation with rules, lists, or similar items; excessive devotion to work, with no attention paid to recreation and friendships; limited expression of warm emotions; reluctance to delegate work and the demand that others submit exactly to his or her way of doing things; and miserliness.

paranoid Characterized by a pervasive distrust and suspiciousness of others such that their motives are interpreted as malevolent. This distrust is shown in many ways, including unreasonable expectation of exploitation or harm by others; questioning without justification the loyalty or trustworthiness of friends or associates; reading demeaning or threatening meanings into benign remarks or events; having a tendency to bear grudges and be unforgiving of insults or injuries; or experiencing unfounded, recurrent suspiciousness about fidelity of his or her sexual partner.

passive-aggressive Cited in older literature and characterized by unassertive resistance and general obstructiveness in response to the expectations of others. Some of these actions are procrastination; postponement of completion of routine tasks; sulkiness, irritability, or argumentiveness if asked to do something he or she does not want to do, and then working unreasonably slowly and inefficiently; or avoidance of obligations by claiming to have forgotten.

schizoid Characterized by detachment from social relationships and restricted emotional range in interpersonal settings. Some examples are that the person neither desires nor enjoys close relationships, prefers solitary activities, appears indifferent to praise or criticism, has no (or only one) close friends or confidants, and is emotionally cold or detached.

schizotypal Characterized by a combination of discomfort with and reduced capacity for close relationships, and cognitive or perceptual distortions and eccentricities of behavior. Possible manifestations include odd beliefs or *magical thinking* inconsistent with cultural norms; unusual perceptual experiences including bodily *illusions;* odd thinking and speech; no (or only one) close friends because of lack of desire, discomfort with others, or eccentricities; and persisting, excessive social *anxiety* that tends to be associated with paranoid fears rather than negative judgments about oneself. Some studies suggest that schizotypal personality disorder might more properly be considered a part of a schizophrenia spectrum disorder.

persuasion A therapeutic approach based on direct suggestion and guidance intended to influence favorably patients' attitudes, behaviors, and goals.

pervasive developmental disorders In DSM-IV, this group includes *autistic disorder, Rett's disorder,* and childhood *disintegrative disorder.* Some authorities also include *Asperger's disorder* within this group.

perversion An imprecise term used to designate sexual variance. See *paraphilia.*

petit mal See *epilepsy.*

PGY-1 See *internship.*

phallic phase See *psychosexual development.*

phantom limb A phenomenon frequently experienced by amputees in which sensations, often painful, appear to originate in the amputated extremity.

pharmacokinetics The study of the process and rates of drug distribution, metabolism, and disposition in the organism.

phase-of-life problem Difficulty in adapting to a particular developmental phase that is not due to a *mental disorder*. Some examples are entering school, leaving parental control, and starting a new career. Other examples are the changes involved in marriage, divorce, or retirement.

phencyclidine (PCP) See TABLE OF COMMONLY ABUSED DRUGS.

phencyclidine use disorders In DSM-IV, this group includes phencyclidine (or related substance) dependence, phencyclidine abuse, phencyclidine intoxication, phencyclidine delirium, phencyclidine psychotic disorder with delusions or hallucinations, phencyclidine mood disorder, and phencyclidine anxiety disorder.

phenomenology The study of occurrences or happenings in their own right, rather than from the point of view of inferred causes; specifically, the theory that behavior is determined not by external reality as it can be described objectively in physical terms, but rather by the way in which the subject perceives that reality at any moment. See also *existential psychiatry*.

phenothiazine derivatives A *neuroleptic* subgroup of *psychotropic* drugs that, chemically, have in common a phenothiazine configuration (i.e., phenyl rings and heterocyclic ring containing nitrogen and sulfur) but differ from one another through variations in side chains. See TABLE OF DRUGS USED IN PSYCHIATRY.

phenotype The observable attributes of an individual; the physical manifestations of the *genotype*.

phenylketonuria (PKU) A genetic, metabolic disturbance characterized by an inability to convert phenylalanine to tyrosine. Results in the abnormal accumulation of chemicals that interfere with brain development. Treatable by diet when detected in early infancy. If untreated, *mental retardation* results. Also known as phenylpyruvic oligophrenia.

phobia *Fear* cued by the presence or anticipation of a specific object or situation, exposure to which almost invariably provokes an immediate *anxiety* response or *panic attack* even though the subject recognizes that the fear is excessive or unreasonable. The phobic stimulus is avoided or endured with marked distress. In earlier psychoanalytic literature, phobia was called *anxiety hysteria*.

Two types of phobia have been differentiated: specific phobia (simple phobia) and social phobia. Specific phobia is subtyped on the basis of the object feared. The natural environment (animals, insects, storms, water, etc.); blood, injection, or injury; situations (cars, airplanes, heights, tunnels, etc.); and other situations that may lead to choking, vomiting, or contracting an illness are all specific phobias.

In social phobia (social anxiety disorder), the persistent fear is of social situations that might expose one to scrutiny by others and induce one to act in a way or show anxiety symptoms that will be humiliating or embarrassing. Avoidance may be limited to one or only a few situations, or it may occur in most social situations. Performing in front of others or social interactions may be the focus of concern. It is sometimes difficult to distinguish between social phobia and *agoraphobia* when social avoidance accompanies panic attacks. *Avoidant disorder* has been used to refer to social phobia occurring in childhood and adolescence.

Some of the common phobias are (add "abnormal fear of" to each entry):

achluophobia Darkness

acrophobia Heights

agoraphobia Open spaces or leaving the familiar setting of the home

ailurophobia Cats

algophobia Pain

androphobia Men
autophobia Being alone or solitude
bathophobia Depths
claustrophobia Closed spaces
cynophobia Dogs
demophobia Crowds
erythrophobia Blushing; sometimes used to refer to the blushing itself
gynophobia Women
hypnophobia Sleep
mysophobia Dirt and germs
panphobia Everything
pedophobia Children
xenophobia Strangers

phonological disorder Articulation disorder; a *communication disorder* characterized by failure in developmentally expected speech that is appropriate for age or dialect. Speech sounds may be omitted, substituted, or distorted, as in saying "w" for "r" or "f" for "th."

phrenology Theory of the relationship between the structure of the skull and mental traits.

phylogenetic Pertaining to the development of the species. Contrast with *ontogenetic.*

pia mater The innermost of the meninges; a delicate fibrous membrane closely enveloping the brain and spinal cord.

Piaget, Jean (1896–1980) Swiss *psychologist* noted for his theoretical concepts of and research on the mental development of children. See also *cognitive development.*

piblokto See *culture-specific syndromes.*

pica A feeding and eating disorder of infancy or early childhood characterized by developmentally inappropriate, persistent, or recurring eating of nonnutritive substances.

Pick's disease A presenile degenerative disease of the brain, possibly hereditary, affecting the cerebral cortex focally, particularly the frontal lobes. *Symptoms* include intellectual deterioration, emotional instability, and loss of social adjustment. See also *Alzheimer's disease.*

piloerection Gooseflesh; it may be a prominent sign in opiod withdrawal.

Pinel, Philippe (1745–1826) French physician-reformer who was a pioneer in abolishing the use of restraints for mentally ill persons.

piperazine See TABLE OF DRUGS USED IN PSYCHIATRY.

piperidine See TABLE OF DRUGS USED IN PSYCHIATRY.

placebo A material without pharmacological activity but identical in appearance to an active drug. Used in pharmacological research as a method of determining the actual effects of the drug being tested. See also LIST OF RESEARCH TERMS.

placebo effect The production or enhancement of psychological or physical effects using pharmacologically inactive substances administered under circumstances in which suggestion leads the subject to believe a particular effect will occur. See also LIST OF RESEARCH TERMS.

plaques Certain areas of the brain that have undergone a specific form of degeneration. Senile plaques (neuritic plaques) consist of a central amyloid core surrounded by a less densely staining zone composed of abnormal *neurons,* with many axonal and dendritic processes and masses of paired helical filaments. In *Alzheimer's disease,* they are particularly dense in the amygdaloid complex and the *hippocampus.* The relationship between the abnormal protein fibers inside neurons (the paired helical filaments) and those outside the cells (i.e., amyloid) is currently unknown. The AD-DP gene, which codes for the beta-amyloid protein that accumulates in the blood vessel walls and in the neuronal tissue in both Alzheimer's and aged Down brains, maps to *chromosome 21.*

plasma level See *blood levels.*

play therapy A treatment technique utilizing the child's play as a medium for expression and communication between patient and therapist.

pleasure principle The psychoanalytic concept (see *psychoanalysis*) that people instinctually seek to avoid pain and discomfort and strive for gratification and pleasure. In personality development theory, the pleasure principle antedates and subsequently comes in conflict with the *reality principle.*

polyphagia Pathological overeating. Also known as bulimia.

polysomnography The all-night recording of a variety of physiological parameters (e.g., brain waves, eye movements, muscle tonus, respiration, heart rate, penile tumescence) in order to diagnose *sleep*-related disorders.

polysubstance use disorders DSM-IV recognizes one disorder, polysubstance dependence, characterized by use of at least three different substances (not including nicotine or caffeine) for 6 months or more during which time no single substance has predominated.

"poppers" See *nitrites.*

porphyria A metabolic disorder characterized by the excretion of porphyrins in the urine and accompanied by attacks of abdominal pain, peripheral neuropathy, and a variety of mental symptoms. Some types are precipitated by *barbiturates* and alcohol.

positive schizophrenia See *schizophrenia.*

positive symptoms See *schizophrenia.*

positron-emission tomography (PET) A *brain-imaging* technique that permits one to evaluate regional metabolic differences by looking at radio-isotope distribution. By using positron-emitting isotopes of glucose, oxygen, neurotransmitters, or drugs, one can localize sites of increased (or decreased) metabolic turnover, receptor findings, or blood flow in a wide variety of neurologic or psychiatric conditions. The visual display is similar to that in *computed tomography (CT)*.

possession See *trance disorder, dissociative.*

postconcussional disorder A history of head trauma with loss of consciousness occurring within 4 weeks after the trauma and followed by somatic complaints (headache, dizziness, noise intolerance), emotional changes (irritability, *depression, anxiety*), difficulty in concentration, *insomnia,* and reduced tolerance to alcohol. Physical examination and laboratory tests give evidence of cerebral damage.

posthallucinogen perception disorder *Flashback;* following cessation of use of a hallucinogen, reexperiencing one or more of the perceptual *symptoms* that had been experienced while using the hallucinogen. Some examples are the *illusion* of objects changing shape, false perceptions of movement in the peripheral field of vision, flashes or intensification of colors, or trails of images of moving objects. See *intoxication, hallucinogen.*

postpartum psychosis An inexact term for any *psychosis* (organic or functional) occurring within 90 days after childbirth.

posttraumatic stress disorder (PTSD) An *anxiety disorder* in which exposure to an exceptional mental or physical stessor is followed, sometimes immediately and sometimes not until 3 months or more after the stress, by persistent reexperiencing of the event, avoidance of stimuli associated with the trauma or numbing of general responsiveness, and manifestations of increased arousal. The trauma typically includes experiencing, witnessing, or confronting an event that involves actual or threatened death or injury, or a threat to the physical integrity of oneself or others, with an immediate reaction of intense fear, helplessness, or horror.

Reexperiencing the trauma may take several forms: recurrent, intrusive, and distressing recollections (images, thoughts, or perceptions) of the event; recurrent distressing dreams of the event; sudden feeling as if the event were recurring or being relived (including dissociative flashback episodes); or intense psychological distress or physiological reactivity if exposed to internal or external cues that symbolize or resemble some part of the event.

The affected person tries to avoid thoughts or feelings associated with the event and anything that might arouse recollection of it. There may be *amnesia* for an important aspect of the trauma. The person may lose interest in significant activities, feel detached or estranged from others, or have a sense of a foreshortened future.

The person may have difficulty falling or staying asleep, be irritable or have angry outbursts, experience problems concentrating, and have an exaggerated startle response.

postural tremor, medication-induced Fine shaking when attempting to maintain a posture that develops in association with the use of medications such as *lithium, antidepressant drugs,* and valproate.

posturing See *catatonic behavior.*

potency The male's ability to carry out sexual relations. Often used to refer specifically to the capacity to have and maintain adequate erection of the penis during sexual intercourse. See also *impotence.*

poverty of speech Restriction in the amount of speech; spontaneous speech and replies to questions range from brief and unelaborated to monosyllabic or no response at all. When the amount of speech is adequate, there may be a poverty of content if the answer is vague or if there is a substitution of stereotyped or obscure phrases for meaningful responses.

preconscious Thoughts that are not in immediate awareness but that can be recalled by *conscious* effort.

pregenital In *psychoanalysis,* refers to the period of early childhood before the genitals have begun to exert the predominant influence in the organization or patterning of sexual behavior. Oral and anal influences predominate during this period. See also *psychosexual development.*

premature ejaculation Undesired ejaculation occurring immediately before or very early in sexual intercourse. One of the *orgasm disorders.*

premenstrual dysphoric disorder Noted in DSM-IV as an example of a *depressive disorder not otherwise specified.* Characteristics are rapidly changing feelings or persistent and marked anger, *anxiety,* or tension; depressed *mood* with feelings of hopelesness or self-deprecating thought; and many other *symptoms* such as lethargy, difficulty in concentrating, overeating or food cravings, *insomnia* or *hypersomnia,* breast tenderness or swelling, headaches, weight gain, increased sensitivity to rejection and avoidance of social activities, or increased interpersonal conflicts. The syndrome occurs in as many as 5% of menstruating women, with symptoms concentrated in the week before and a few days after the onset of menses.

presenile dementia A *dementia* of the Alzheimer type beginning before age 65. See also *Alzheimer's disease; Pick's disease.*

pressured speech Rapid, accelerated, frenzied speech. Sometimes it exceeds the ability of the vocal musculature to articulate, leading to jumbled and cluttered speech; at other times it exceeds the ability of the listener to comprehend as the speech expresses a *flight of ideas* (as in *mania*) or unintelligible jargon. See also *logorrhea.*

prevalence Frequency of a disorder, used particularly in *epidemiology* to denote the total number of cases existing within a unit of population at a given time or over a specified period.

prevention (preventive psychiatry) In traditional medical usage, the prevention or prophylaxis of a disorder. In *community psychiatry,* the meaning of prevention encompasses the amelioration, control, and limitation of disease. Prevention is often categorized as follows:

  primary prevention Measures implemented to prevent the occurrence of a *mental disorder* (e.g., by nutrition, substitute parents, etc.).

  secondary prevention Measures implemented to limit an existing disease process (e.g., through early case-finding and treatment).

  tertiary prevention Measures implemented to reduce impairment or disability following development of a disorder (e.g., through *rehabilitation* programs).

primal scene In psychoanalytic theory (see *psychoanalysis*), the real or fancied observation by the child of parental or other heterosexual intercourse.

primal scream therapy See *experiential therapy.*

primary care physician Usually a general practitioner or specialist in family practice, internal medicine, pediatrics, or, occasionally, obstetrics and gynecology who serves as an initial contact for patients in managed health care systems.

primary degenerative dementia See *Alzheimer's disease.*

primary diagnosis The condition established after study to be the most severe condition for which the patient receives treatment.

primary gain The relief from emotional *conflict* and the freedom from *anxiety* achieved by a *defense mechanism.* Contrast with *secondary gain.*

primary process In psychoanalytic theory (see *psychoanalysis*), the generally unorganized mental activity characteristic of the *unconscious*. This activity is marked by the free discharge of energy and excitation without regard to the demands of environment, reality, or logic. See also *secondary process*.

Prince, Morton (1854–1929) American *psychiatrist* and *neurologist* known for his work on *multiple personality*.

principal diagnosis The condition established after study to be chiefly responsible for the admission of the patient to the hospital or for outpatient treatment.

prison psychosis See *Ganser's syndrome*.

privileged communication Information imparted by a patient or client within the context of a professional relationship with a practitioner (i.e., physician, lawyer) that is immune to disclosure without the patient's or client's expressed permission.

problem solving A specific form of intellectual activity used when a person faces a situation that cannot be handled in terms of past learning. Problem-solving strategies are considered crucial in any psychotherapeutic endeavor.

problem-oriented record A simple conceptual framework to expedite and improve medical records. It contains four logically sequenced sections: the database, the problem list, plans, and follow-up.

process schizophrenia See under *schizophrenia*.

prodrome (precursor) An early or premonitory *symptom* or set of symptoms of a disease or a disorder.

professional standards review organization (PSRO) A physician-sponsored organization charged with comprehensive and ongoing review of services provided under Medicare, Medicaid, and maternal and child health programs. The object of this review is to determine for purposes of reimbursement under these programs whether services are medically necessary;

provided in accordance with professional criteria, norms, and standards; and, in the case of institutional services, rendered in appropriate settings. See also *peer review organization (PRO).*

prognosis The prediction of the future course of an illness.

projection A *defense mechanism,* operating unconsciously (see *unconscious*), in which what is emotionally unacceptable in the self is unconsciously rejected and attributed (projected) to others.

projective identification A term introduced by Melanie *Klein* to refer to the *unconscious* process of *projection* of one or more parts of the self or of the internal object into another person (such as the mother). What is projected may be an intolerable, painful, or dangerous part of the self or object (the *bad object*). It may also be a valued aspect of the self or object (the good object) that is projected into the other person for safekeeping. The other person is changed by the projection and is dealt with as though he or she is in fact characterized by the aspects of the self that have been projected.

projective tests Psychological diagnostic tests in which the test material is unstructured so that any response will reflect a *projection* of some aspect of the subject's underlying *personality* and *psychopathology.* See also TABLE OF PSYCHOLOGICAL TESTS.

prolactin A hormone secreted by the anterior pituitary that promotes lactation in the female and may stimulate testosterone secretion in the male. Prolactin secretion is in part controlled by inhibiting and releasing factors in the brain. Because *dopamine* is involved in the brain's inhibition of prolactin secretion, the measurement of serum prolactin has been proposed as a way of judging the efficacy of specific antipsychotic drugs that act by blocking dopamine's effects.

proxy symptoms See *factitious disorders.*

pseudocyesis Included in DSM-IV as one of the *somatoform disorders*. It is characterized by a false belief of being pregnant and by the occurrence of signs of being pregnant, such as abdominal enlargement, breast engorgement, and labor pains.

pseudodementia A *syndrome* in which *dementia* is mimicked or caricatured by a functional psychiatric illness. *Symptoms* and response of *mental status examination* questions are similar to those found in verified cases of *dementia*. In pseudodementia, the chief diagnosis to be considered in the differential is *depression* in an older person vs. cognitive deterioration on the basis of organic brain disease. See also *Ganser's syndrome*.

psyche The mind.

psychedelic A term applied to any of several drugs that may induce *hallucinations* and altered mental states, including the production of distortions of time, sound, color, and so forth. Among the more commonly used psychedelics are *LSD, marijuana, mescaline,* and psilocybin. See also TABLE OF COMMONLY ABUSED DRUGS.

psychiatric illness See *mental disorder*.

Psychiatric News The bimonthly newspaper of the *American Psychiatric Association*.

psychiatric nurse Any nurse employed in a psychiatric hospital or other psychiatric setting who has special training and experience in the management of psychiatric patients. Sometimes the term is used to denote only those nurses who have a master's degree in psychiatric nursing.

psychiatric social work A specialty of *social work* that is concerned with the prevention of *mental illness,* the treatment and rehabilitation of mentally ill patients, and the prevention of relapse. Particular attention is given to familial, environmental, cultural, and other social factors that may be involved in the development, continuation, or recurrence of mental illness and in the patient's response to treatment.

psychiatrist A licensed physician who specializes in the diagnosis, treatment, and prevention of mental and emotional disorders. Training encompasses a medical degree and 4 years or more of approved postgraduate training. For those who wish to enter a subspecialty such as *child psychiatry, geriatric psychiatry, psychoanalysis,* administration, addiction psychiatry, and the like, additional training is required.

psychiatry The medical science that deals with the origin, diagnosis, prevention, and treatment of *mental disorders.*

psychic determinism See *determinism.*

psychoactive substance use disorders See *drug dependence.*

psychoanalysis A theory of the *psychology* of human development and behavior, a method of research, and a system of *psychotherapy,* originally developed by *Freud.* Through analysis of *free associations* and *interpretation* of dreams, *emotions* and behavior are traced to the influence of repressed instinctual *drives* and defenses against them in the *unconscious.* Psychoanalytic treatment seeks to eliminate or diminish the undesirable effects of unconscious *conflicts* by making the *analysand* aware of their existence, origin, and inappropriate expression in current emotions and behavior. See also OUTLINE OF SCHOOLS OF PSYCHIATRY.

psychoanalyst A person, usually a *psychiatrist,* who has had training in *psychoanalysis* and who employs the techniques of psychoanalytic theory in the treatment of patients.

psychoanalytically oriented psychotherapy A form of *psychotherapy* that employs a variety of techniques, some of which are close to the practice of *psychoanalysis* (e.g., use of clarification and interpretation), and others that are quite different (e.g., the use of suggestion, reassurance, and advice giving). It is now generally seen as existing on a continuum with psychoanalysis and is often termed psychoanalytic psychotherapy.

psychobiology A school of psychiatric thought that views biological, psychological, and social life experiences of a person as an integrated unit. Associated with Adolf *Meyer,* who introduced the term in the United States in 1915. See also OUTLINE OF SCHOOLS OF PSYCHIATRY.

psychodrama A technique of *group psychotherapy* conceived and practiced by the late J. L. Moreno, M.D. (1890–1974), in which individuals express their own or assigned emotional problems in dramatization.

psychodynamics The systematized knowledge and theory of human behavior and its motivation, the study of which depends largely upon the functional significance of *emotion.* Psychodynamics recognizes the role of *unconscious* motivation in human behavior. The science of psychodynamics assumes that one's behavior is determined by past experience, genetic endowment, and current reality.

psychoendocrinology The study of the psychological effects of neuroendocrinological activity. For example, it is known that the release and inhibition of pituitary hormones are mediated in part by brain monoamines, disorders of which have been implicated in the pathogenesis of various psychiatric illnesses.

psychogenesis Production or causation of a *symptom* or illness by mental or psychic factors as opposed to organic ones.

psychogenic amnesia See *amnesia.*

psychogenic fugue See *fugue.*

psychogenic pain disorder In DSM-IV, called pain disorder associated with psychological factors and classified as a *somatoform disorder;* pain for which adequate physical findings are absent and for which there is evidence that psychological factors play a causal role.

psychohistory An approach to history that examines events within a psychological framework.

psychoimmunology The study of the connection between the brain and emotions and the immune system.

psycholinguistics The study of factors affecting activities involved in communicating and comprehending verbal information. See also *kinesics.*

psychological autopsy Postmortem evaluations of the *psychodynamics* leading to a person's *suicide.*

psychological tests See TABLE OF PSYCHOLOGICAL TESTS.

psychologist A person who holds a degree in *psychology* from an accredited program. Providers of psychological services are licensed under applicable state law, whereas those who teach or do research are usually exempt from licensure requirements.

psychology An academic discipline, a profession, and a science dealing with the study of mental processes and behavior of people and animals.

psychology, analytic See *analytic psychology; Jung.*

psychology, individual See *individual psychology; Adler.*

psychometry The science of testing and measuring mental and psychological ability, efficiency potentials, and functioning, including psychopathological components (see *psychopathology*). See also TABLE OF PSYCHOLOGICAL TESTS.

psychomotor Referring to combined physical and mental activity.

psychomotor agitation Excessive motor activity associated with a feeling of inner tension. When severe, agitation may involve shouting and loud complaining. The activity is usually nonproductive and repetitious, and consists of such behavior as pacing, wringing of hands, and inability to sit still.

psychomotor retardation A generalized slowing of physical and emotional reactions. Specifically, the slowing of movements such as eye blinking; frequently seen in *depression*.

psychoneurosis See *neurosis*.

psychopathic personality Antisocial personality disorder. See *personality disorder*.

psychopathology The study of the significant causes and processes in the development of *mental disorders*. Also the manifestations of mental disorders.

psychopharmacology The study of the effects of psychoactive drugs on behavior in both animals and people. Clinical psychopharmacology more specifically includes both the study of drug effects in patients and the expert use of drugs in the treatment of psychiatric conditions.

psychophysiological disorders A group of disorders characterized by physical *symptoms* that are affected by emotional factors and involve a single organ system, usually under *autonomic nervous system* control. Symptoms are caused by physiological changes that normally accompany certain emotional states, but the changes are more intense and sustained. Frequently called *psychosomatic* disorders. These disorders are usually named and classified according to the organ system involved (e.g., gastrointestinal, respiratory). In DSM-IV, such cases would be diagnosed as psychological factors affecting a *general medical condition*. The specific physical condition is diagnosed and recorded separately. In cases where there is no diagnosable physical condition, some other disorder may be cited. See *autonomic arousal disorder*.

psychosexual development A series of stages from infancy to adulthood, relatively fixed in time, determined by the interaction between a person's biological *drives* and the environment. With resolution of this interaction, a balanced, reality-oriented development takes place; with disturbance, *fixation* and *conflict* ensue. This disturbance may remain latent or give rise to characterological or behavioral disorders. In classical psychoanalytic psychology, the stages of development are as follows:

oral The earliest of the stages of infantile psychosexual development, lasting from birth to 12 months or longer. Usually subdivided into two stages: the oral *erotic,* relating to the pleasurable experience of sucking; and the oral sadistic, associated with aggressive biting. Both oral eroticism and *sadism* continue into adult life in disguised and sublimated forms, such as the character traits of demandingness or pessimism. Oral conflict, as a general and pervasive influence, might underlie the psychological determinants of addictive disorders, *depression,* and some functional psychotic disorders.

anal The period of *pregenital* psychosexual development, usually from 1 to 3 years, in which the child has particular interest and concern with the process of defecation and the sensations connected with the anus. The pleasurable part of the experience is termed anal eroticism. See also *anal character.*

phallic The period, from about 2½ to 6 years, during which sexual interest, curiosity, and pleasurable experience in boys center on the penis, and in girls, to a lesser extent, the clitoris.

oedipal Overlapping some with the phallic stage, this phase (ages 4 to 6) represents a time of inevitable conflict between the child and parents. The child must desexualize the relationship to both parents in order to retain affectionate kinship with both of them. The process is accomplished by the internalization of the images of both parents, thereby giving more definite shape to the child's personality. With this internalization largely completed, the regulation of self-esteem and moral behavior comes from within.

psychosexual dysfunction A disorder characterized by an inhibition in sexual desire; sexual excitement, *orgasm, premature ejaculation, dyspareunia,* or *vaginismus* may be present. In DSM-IV, called *sexual and gender identity disorders* to reflect more accurately the fact that a biogenic component is often present.

psychosis A severe *mental disorder* characterized by gross impairment in *reality testing,* typically shown by *delusions, hallucinations,* disorganized speech, or disorganized or *catatonic behavior.* Persons with these disorders are termed psychotic. Among these illnesses are *schizophrenia, delusional disorders,* some secondary or symptomatic disorders ("organic psychoses"), and some *mood disorders.*

psychosocial development Progressive interaction between a person and the environment through stages beginning in infancy, as described by *Erikson.* Specific developmental tasks involving social relations and the role of social reality are faced by a person at phase-specific developmental points. The early tasks parallel stages of *psychosexual development;* the later tasks extend through adulthood. Successful and unsuccessful solutions to each task are listed below with the corresponding chronological period and psychosexual stage where applicable. See also *cognitive development.*

Task and solutions	Chronological period	Psychosexual stage
Trust vs. mistrust	Infancy	Oral
Autonomy vs. shame, doubt	Early childhood (toddler)	Anal
Initiative vs. guilt	Preschool	Phallic (oedipal)

Task and solutions	Chronological period	Psychosexual stage
Industry vs. inferiority	School-age	Latency
Identity vs. identity diffusion	Adolescence	
Intimacy vs. isolation	Young adulthood	Genital
Generativity vs. self-absorption	Adulthood	
Integrity vs. despair	Mature age	

psychosomatic Referring to the constant and insepa-
rable interaction of the *psyche* (mind) and the *soma*
(body). Most commonly used to refer to illnesses in
which the manifestations are primarily physical but
with at least a partial emotional etiology. See also
psychophysiological disorders.

psychosurgery Surgical intervention to sever fibers
connecting one part of the brain with another or to
remove or destroy brain tissue with the intent of
modifying or altering severe disturbances of behavior,
thought content, or *mood.* Such surgery may also be
undertaken for the relief of intractable pain. See
lobotomy.

psychotherapist A person trained to practice *psychotherapy.*

psychotherapy A process in which a person who
wishes to relieve *symptoms* or resolve problems in
living or is seeking personal growth enters into an
implicit or explicit contract to interact in a prescribed
way with a *psychotherapist.* See also *brief psychotherapy.*

psychotic depression See *depression with psychotic features* and *melancholia.*

psychotic disorder, brief A transient disorder with duration limited from a few hours to 1 month and an eventual return to full functioning. *Symptoms* during the episode indicate impaired *reality testing* that is not culturally sanctioned, *delusions, hallucinations,* disorganized speech, or disorganized or *catatonic behavior.* When such symptoms are a reaction to marked stressors, they are sometimes labeled brief reactive psychosis.

psychotic disorder due to a general medical condition Prominent *hallucinations* or *delusions* that develop in relation to some general medical condition. In older classifications, such disorders were termed organic brain syndromes or secondary psychotic disorders.

psychotic disorder, shared Induced psychotic disorder; for example, person A develops a *delusion* in the context of a close relationship with person B, who has an already established delusion. The delusion in person A is similar in content to person B's delusion. One example is folie à deux.

psychotic disorder, substance-induced See *substance-induced psychotic disorder.*

psychotomimetic Literally, mimicking a *psychosis.* Used to refer to certain drugs such as *LSD* or *mescaline* that may produce psychotic-like states.

psychotropic A term used to describe drugs that have a special action upon the *psyche.* See also TABLE OF DRUGS USED IN PSYCHIATRY.

PTSD *Posttraumatic stress disorder.*

pyromania Firesetting; an *impulse control disorder* consisting of deliberate and purposeful firesetting on more than one occasion. As in other disorders of impulse control, an increasing sense of tension or affective arousal immediately precedes the action, and its completion brings a sense of intense pleasure, gratification, or relief.

Q

Q-sort See LIST OF RESEARCH TERMS.

quality assurance Activities and programs intended to assure the standard of care in a defined medical setting or program. Such programs must include educational components intended to remedy identified deficiencies in quality.

R

random A statistical term that denotes accuracy by chance or without attention to selection or planning. See also *random sample* in LIST OF RESEARCH TERMS.

Rank, Otto (1884–1939) Viennese lay *psychoanalyst* and early follower of *Freud. The Trauma of Birth,* his major book, was published in 1924. He emigrated to the United States in 1935 and strongly influenced the Philadelphia Child Guidance Center and the University of Pennsylvania School of Social Work.

rape Sexual assault; forced sexual intercourse without the partner's consent.

rapid cycling Referring to *bipolar disorder* in which four or more episodes of mood disturbance (*manic, hypomanic,* or major depressive episode) occur within 1 year.

rapport The feeling of harmonious accord and mutual responsiveness that contributes to the patient's confidence in the therapist and willingness to work cooperatively. To be distinguished from *transference,* which is *unconscious.*

rational-emotive psychotherapy See *experiential therapy.*

rationalization A *defense mechanism,* operating unconsciously, in which an individual attempts to justify or make consciously tolerable by plausible means, feelings or behavior that otherwise would be intolerable. Not to be confused with conscious evasion or dissimulation. See also *projection.*

Ray, Isaac (1807–1881) A founder of the *American Psychiatric Association* whose *Treatise on the Medical Jurisprudence of Insanity* was the pioneering American work in *forensic psychiatry.*

reaction formation A *defense mechanism,* operating unconsciously, in which a person adopts *affects,* ideas, and behaviors that are the opposites of impulses harbored either consciously or unconsciously (see *conscious; unconscious*). For example, excessive moral zeal may be a reaction to strong but repressed asocial impulses.

reactive attachment disorder See *attachment disorder, reactive.*

reactive depression See *depression.*

reactive psychosis, brief See *psychotic disorder, brief.*

reading disorder One of the *academic skills disorders,* characterized by impaired reading accuracy or comprehension that interferes significantly with academic performance or activities of living that require reading skills. Reading achievement is substantially below that expected given the subject's age, measured intelligence, and age-appropriate education.

reality principle In psychoanalytic theory (see *psychoanalysis*), the concept that the *pleasure principle,* which represents the claims of instinctual wishes, is normally modified by the demands and requirements of the external world. In fact, the reality principle may still work on behalf of the pleasure principle but reflects compromises and allows for the postponement of gratification to a more appropriate time. The reality principle usually becomes more prominent in the course of development but may be weak in certain psychiatric illnesses and undergo strengthening during treatment.

reality testing The ability to evaluate the external world objectively and to differentiate adequately between it and the internal world. Falsification of reality, as with massive *denial* or *projection,* indicates a severe disturbance of *ego* functioning and/or of the perceptual and memory processes upon which it is partly based. See also *psychosis.*

reality therapy See *experiential therapy.*

recall The process of bringing a memory into consciousness (see *conscious*). Recall is often used to refer to the recollection of facts, events, and feelings that occurred in the immediate past.

receptive language disorder See *communication disorders.*

receptor A specialized area on a nerve membrane, a blood vessel, or a muscle that receives the chemical stimulation that activates or inhibits the nerve, blood vessel, or muscle.

reciprocal inhibition In *behavior therapy,* the hypothesis that if *anxiety*-provoking stimuli occur simultaneously with the inhibition of anxiety (e.g., relaxation), the bond between those stimuli and the anxiety will be weakened.

recurrent brief depressive disorder See *depressive disorders.*

reductionism See *epigenetics.*

reference, delusion of (idea of) See *ideas of reference.*

regional cerebral blood flow (rCBF) A measurement obtained by using a noninvasive technique such as radioactive xenon to chart brain blood flow. See also *brain imaging.*

regression Partial or symbolic return to earlier patterns of reacting or thinking. Manifested in a wide variety of circumstances such as normal *sleep,* play, physical illness, and in many *mental disorders.*

rehabilitation In *psychiatry,* the methods and techniques used to achieve maximum functioning and optimum adjustment for the patient and to prevent relapses or recurrences of illness; sometimes termed *tertiary prevention* (see under *prevention*).

Reich, Wilhelm (1897–1957) Austrian *psychoanalyst* who emigrated to the United States in 1939; noted for his emphasis on the necessity of free expression of sexual *libido* during orgasm (orgone) as a cure for *neurosis.*

Reik, Theodor (1888–1969) Viennese *psychoanalyst* and early follower of *Freud* who made valuable contributions to psychoanalysis on the subjects of religion, *masochism,* and therapeutic technique.

reinforcement The strengthening of a response by reward or avoidance of punishment. This process is central in *operant conditioning.*

relatedness Sense of *sympathy* and *empathy* with others.

relational problems Family and partner difficulties, not necessarily due to *mental disorder* but often the focus of consultation or treatment. DSM-IV specifies parent-child relational problem (with physical or sexual abuse or neglect of child, inadequate parental discipline, parental overprotection, or communication problems); partner relational problem (with negative or distorted communication); and sibling relational problem.

REM latency The time lag between *sleep* onset (stage 2 sleep) and the first REM period minus any awake time. See *sleep*.

REM sleep Rapid eye movement *sleep*.

reminiscence A normal, universal process of life review in an elderly person prompted in part by the realization of approaching death. The person reviews past life and conflicts and possibilities for their resolution. *Depression, anxiety,* regret, and despair may be present.

remission Abatement of an illness.

repetition compulsion In psychoanalytic theory (see *psychoanalysis*), the impulse to reenact earlier emotional experiences. Considered by *Freud* to be more fundamental than the *pleasure principle.* Defined by *Jones* in the following way: "The blind impulse to repeat earlier experiences and situations quite irrespective of any advantage that doing so might bring from a pleasure-pain point of view."

repression A *defense mechanism,* operating unconsciously, that banishes unacceptable ideas, fantasies, *affects,* or impulses from consciousness or that keeps out of consciousness what has never been *conscious.* Although not subject to voluntary recall, the repressed material may emerge in disguised form. Often confused with the conscious mechanism of *suppression.*

reserpine An alkaloid (of Rauwolfia serpentina) used for treatment of hypertension and formerly used for *psychosis* or other psychiatric disorders.

resident A physician who is in graduate training to qualify as a specialist in a particular field of medicine, such as *psychiatry.* The *American Board of Psychiatry and Neurology, Inc.* requires 4 years of postgraduate training in an approved facility to qualify for board examination in psychiatry.

residential treatment facility See *halfway house.*

residual A term describing the phase of an illness that occurs after remission of the florid *symptoms* or the full *syndrome*. The remaining symptoms are called residua.

residual schizophrenia See *schizophrenia.*

resistance One's *conscious* or *unconscious* psychological defense against bringing *repressed* (unconscious) thoughts into *conscious* awareness.

respondent conditioning (classical conditioning, Pavlovian conditioning) Elicitation of a response by a stimulus that normally does not elicit that response. The response is one that is mediated primarily by the *autonomic nervous system* (such as salivation or a change in heart rate). A previously neutral stimulus is repeatedly presented just before an unconditioned stimulus that normally elicits that response. When the response subsequently occurs in the presence of the previously neutral stimulus, it is called a conditioned response, and the previously neutral stimulus, a conditioned stimulus.

restricted affect See *affect.*

restricting type See *anorexia nervosa.*

RET See *experiential therapy.*

retardation See *retardation, mental; psychomotor retardation.*

retardation, mental A major group of disorders of infancy, childhood, or adolescence characterized by intellectual functioning that is significantly below average (IQ of 70 or below), manifested before the age of 18 by impaired adaptive functioning (below expected performance for age in such areas as social or daily living skills, communication, and self-sufficiency).

Different levels of severity are recognized:

IQ level	Level of severity
50/55 to 70	Mild
35/40 to 50/55	Moderate
20/25 to 35/40	Severe
below 20/25	Profound

retrograde amnesia See *amnesia*.

retrospective falsification *Unconscious* distortion of past experiences to conform to present emotional needs.

Rett's disorder A *pervasive developmental disorder* characterized by the appearance, between 5 and 48 months of age, of decelerated head growth, loss of previously acquired purposeful hand movements and development of stereotyped hand movements (hand wringing), loss of social engagement (social interaction may develop later), poorly coordinated gait or trunk movements, and impaired expressive and receptive language with severe *psychomotor retardation*. Development during the first 6 months of life appears normal.

rhinorrhea Discharge from the nose; watery rhinorrhea may be a prominent *symptom* in opioid withdrawal.

ribonucleic acid (RNA) A chemical substance involved in cellular protein synthesis. Its structure is coded for by *DNA (deoxyribonucleic acid)*.

rigidity Resistance to change, inflexibility. See *catatonic behavior; extrapyramidal syndrome; parkinsonism*.

ritual A repetitive activity, usually a distorted or stereotyped elaboration of some routine of daily life, employed to relieve *anxiety*. Most commonly seen in *obsessive-compulsive neurosis* (see under *neurosis*).

Rogers, Carl R. (1902–1987) *American psychologist,* a founder of humanistic psychology and known for developing a client-centered approach to *psychotherapy* that permits the patient to take the lead in the focus, pace, and direction of therapy; coined the term "self-actualization" to describe self-discovery and personal growth.

role A pattern of behavior a person acquires or adopts as influenced and expected by significant people in his or her milieu.

rolfing See *experiential therapy.*

Rorschach test See TABLE OF PSYCHOLOGICAL TESTS.

rumination disorder A feeding and eating disorder of infancy consisting of the repeated regurgitation of food in the absence of associated gastrointestinal illness.

Rush, Benjamin (1746–1813) Early American physician, a signer of the Declaration of Independence, and author of the first American book on *psychiatry.* He is known as the father of American psychiatry.

S

SAD Seasonal affective disorder. See *seasonal mood disorder.*

sadism, sexual One of the *paraphilias,* characterized by marked distress over, or acting on, desires to inflict physical or psychological suffering, including humiliation, on the victim.

sadomasochistic relationship Enjoyment of suffering by one person of an interacting couple with a complementary enjoyment in inflicting pain in the other.

satyriasis Pathological or exaggerated sexual drive or excitement in the man. May be of psychological or organic *etiology.* See also *nymphomania* (under *-mania*).

scatologia See *telephone scatologia.*

schizoaffective disorder A *psychotic disorder* in which either a major depressive or a manic episode develops concurrently with the *symptoms* of *schizophrenia;* although *mood* episodes are present for a substantial portion of the psychotic disturbance, there are also periods of *delusions* or *hallucinations* in the absence of prominent mood symptoms.

schizoid personality disorder See *personality disorder.*

schizophrenia A group of idiopathic *psychotic disorders* characterized by both positive and negative *symptoms* associated with disturbance in one or more major areas of functioning such as work, academic development or achievement, interpersonal relations, and self-care. Positive symptoms include *delusions,* which may be bizarre in nature; *hallucinations,* especially auditory; disorganized speech; inappropriate *affect;* and disorganized behavior. Negative symptoms include flat affect, *avolition, alogia,* and **anhedonia.** Duration is variable: ICD-10 requires that continuous signs of the disturbance persist for at least 1 month; DSM-IV requires a minimum of 6 months.

Some of the subtypes are as follows:

paranoid Also termed the positive type. *Delusions* or *hallucinations* dominate the clinical picture.

disorganized (formerly called hebephrenic) Disorganized speech and behavior and inappropriate *affect* dominate the clinical picture; if present at all, *delusions* and *hallucinations* are fragmented.

catatonic Abnormal motor activity dominates the clinical picture. This may take the form of motor immobility, *catalepsy, waxy flexibility,* or *stupor;* extreme *agitation* with purposelessness and excessive motor activity; extreme negativism and resistance or *mutism;* peculiar movements such as posturing, stereotyped movements, prominent mannerisms, or grimacing; and *echolalia* or *echopraxia.*

undifferentiated No one of the above clinical presentations predominates.

residual Persistence of some symptoms but not of sufficient number or intensity to indicate that the patient is in an active phase. The existing symptoms may be only negative (e.g., social isolation, impaired grooming, blunted affect, *poverty of speech,* lack of energy or initiative), but there may also be peculiar behavior, vague and circumstantial speech, odd beliefs or *magical thinking,* or unusual perceptual experiences. Patients who develop *depression* (i.e., depressed mood plus other symptoms of a major depressive episode) during the residual phase are labeled as having postpsychotic depression of schizophrenia.

schizophrenia and other psychotic disorders In DSM-IV, this group includes *schizophrenia, schizophreniform disorder, schizoaffective disorder, delusional disorder, brief psychotic disorder, shared psychotic disorder, psychotic disorder due to a general medical condition,* substance-induced psychotic disorder, and psychotic disorder not otherwise specified. See *secondary disorders.*

schizophreniform disorder Clinical features are the same as those seen in *schizophrenia* but the duration is less than that required for a diagnosis of schizophrenia.

schizotypal personality disorder See *personality disorder.*

school phobia See *separation anxiety disorder.*

schools of psychiatry The various theoretical frames of reference that influence and determine *psychiatrists'* formulations and methods of treatment. Most commonly, the schools explain how psychiatric symptoms or disorders develop, how they interfere with functioning, and how and why they can be altered by therapeutic interventions. See also OUTLINE OF SCHOOLS OF PSYCHIATRY for an arbitrary listing of schools and their founders or leading proponents.

screen memory A consciously tolerable memory that serves as a cover for an associated memory that would be emotionally painful if recalled.

SDAT Senile dementia of the Alzheimer type. See *Alzheimer's disease.*

seasonal mood disorder Seasonal affective disorder (SAD). A mood disorder (*bipolar,* bipolar II, or recurrent major *depressive disorder*) in which there has been a regular temporal relationship between onset or disappearance of the episode and a particular time. For example, a depression regularly appears in the fall or winter, or a regular remission from depression occurs in the spring.

secondary disorder Symptomatic disorder; a *mental disorder* that is due to a *general medical condition* or is induced by a substance. See *organic mental disorder.*

secondary gain The external gain derived from any illness, such as personal attention and service, monetary gains, disability benefits, and release from unpleasant responsibilities. See also *primary gain.*

secondary prevention See *prevention.*

secondary process In psychoanalytic theory (see *psychoanalysis*), mental activity and thinking characteristic of the *ego* and influenced by the demands of the environment. Characterized by organization, systematization, *intellectualization,* and similar processes leading to logical thought and action in adult life. See also *primary process; reality principle.*

sedative A term broadly applied to any agent that quiets, calms, or allays excitement. The term is generally restricted to drugs that are not primarily used to achieve relief from *anxiety.* See also TABLE OF DRUGS USED IN PSYCHIATRY.

sedative/hypnotic/anxiolytic use disorders In DSM-IV, this group includes sedative dependence, sedative abuse, sedative intoxication, sedative withdrawal, sedative delirium, sedative persisting dementia, sedative persisting amnestic disorder, sedative psychotic disorder with delusions or hallucinations, sedative mood disorder, sedative anxiety disorder, sedative sleep disorder, and sedative sexual dysfunction.

selective mutism See *mutism, selective.*

self The psychophysical totality of a person, including both *conscious* and *unconscious* attributes.

self, bipolar See *bipolar self.*

self, grandiose See *grandiose self.*

self psychology A theory of psychoanalytic psychology and a reconceptualization of the psychoanalytic treatment process (see *psychoanalysis*) developed by Heinz *Kohut* (1913–1981) in an effort to transcend the limitations of *ego psychology* that were highlighted by his experience in treating patients with narcissistic and borderline character disorders.

Kohut postulated a separate and nonpathological developmental line for narcissism and described its phase-appropriate needs for self-enhancement and responsivity throughout the life cycle. Self psychology is concerned not with the modulation of drives and the avoidance of conflict, but with the quest for affirmation and actualization in a healthy or enfeebled self.

self-defeating personality disorder Masochistic personality. Its major manifestations include choosing people and situations that lead to disappointment or mistreatment despite the availability of other options; responding to positive personal events with *guilt* or pain-producing behavior; rejecting opportunities for pleasure or enjoyment; or perceiving oneself as undeserving of being treated well. There is continuing controversy over the existence of such an entity.

self-fulfilling prophecy A prediction or supposition of an event or situation that, with frequent repetition, influences a person, the environment, or both to behave as expected by others in this social setting.

self-help groups Troubled people with a common problem who collectively help each other by personal and group support. Examples are *Alcoholics Anonymous* (AA), Gamblers Anonymous (GA), and Narcotics Anonymous (NA).

selfobject In *Kohut's self psychology,* another person (or sometimes an inanimate object or abstract concept) who is experienced as part of the self because of the psychological functions that the other person provides. The other's responses and attitudes are vitally experienced by the developing psyche not only as shapers of the self but as part of the self. The selfobject bridges the gap between *intrapsychic* and sociocultural forces.

senescence A chronological period commonly referred to as old age; characterized by introspection, awareness of death, sense of legacy, and the possibilities of frailty, disability, dependency, and abandonment. Senescence is the result of physiological, psychological, and social forces.

senile dementia A chronic, progressive *dementia* associated with generalized atrophy of the brain involving the death of *neurons* due to unknown causes, although there are several promising theories under study (e.g., autoimmunity, slow virus, cholinergic deficiency). It is not due to aging per se but may be a late form of *Alzheimer's disease*. Deterioration may range from minimal to severe. Senile dementia must be carefully separated from reversible brain syndrome, the latter resulting from many causes.

sensitivity group A group in which members strive to increase self-awareness and understanding of the group's dynamics, as distinct from treatments designed to ameliorate identified, individual, *ego-dystonic* emotional problems.

sensorium Synonymous with consciousness. Includes the special sensory perceptive powers and their central correlation and integration in the brain. A clear sensorium conveys the presence of a reasonably accurate memory together with *orientation* for time, place, and person. See also *mental status*.

sensory deprivation The experience of being cut off from usual external stimuli and the opportunity for *perception*. This may occur experimentally or accidentally in various ways. For example, the loss of hearing or eyesight, physical isolation, or some hospital confinements may lead to disorganized thinking, *delirium, depression, panic, delusions,* and *hallucinations*.

separation anxiety The normal *fear* and apprehension noted in infants when they are removed from the mother (or surrogate mother) or when approached by strangers. Most marked from age 6 to 10 months. In later life, similar reactions may be caused by separation from significant persons or familiar surroundings.

separation anxiety disorder A disorder with onset before the age of 18 consisting of inappropriate *anxiety* concerning separation from home or from persons to whom the child is attached. Among the *symptoms* that may be seen are unrealistic concern about harm befalling or loss of major attachment figures; refusal to go to school (school phobia) in order to stay at home and maintain contact with this figure; refusal to go to *sleep* unless close to this person; clinging; nightmares about the theme of separation; and development of physical symptoms or mood changes (apathy, *depression*) when separation occurs or is anticipated.

separation-individuation Psychological awareness of one's separateness, described by Margaret Mahler as a phase in the mother-child relationship that follows the symbiotic stage. In the separation-individuation stage, the child begins to perceive himself or herself as distinct from the mother and develops a sense of individual identity and an image of the self as object. Mahler described four subphases of the process: differentiation, practicing, rapprochement (i.e., active approach toward the mother, replacing the relative obliviousness to her that prevailed during the practicing period), and separation-individuation proper (i.e., awareness of discrete identity, separateness, and individuality). See also *symbiosis.*

serotonin A *neurotransmitter* with an indole structure found both in peripheral ganglia and in the *central nervous system.* See also *biogenic amines.*

serum levels See *blood levels.*

sexual and gender identity disorders In DSM-IV, this category includes *sexual dysfunctions, paraphilias, gender identity disorder* of childhood, and gender identity disorder of adolescence or adulthood.

sexual arousal disorders One group of *sexual dysfunctions* that includes female sexual arousal disorder and male erectile disorder. Female arousal disorder refers to the inability to attain or maintain an adequate lubrication swelling response of sexual excitement until completion of sexual activity. Male erectile disorder (erectile *impotence*) refers to the inability to attain or maintain an erection until completion of sexual activity.

sexual aversion disorder One of the *sexual desire disorders.*

sexual desire disorders One group of *sexual dysfunctions* that includes hypoactive sexual desire disorder and sexual aversion disorder. Hypoactive sexual desire disorder refers to absent or deficient sexual fantasies and sexual activity that causes the affected person marked distress or interpersonal difficulty. What is judged to be deficient is based on age, sex, the context of the person's life, and similar factors that may affect sexual functioning. Sexual aversion disorder refers to avoidance of and conscious aversion to genital sexual contact with a sexual partner that causes the affected person marked distress or interpersonal difficulty.

sexual deviation See *paraphilias.*

sexual drive One of the two primal drives (the other is the aggressive drive) according to *Freud's* dual-instinct theory.

sexual dysfunctions One of the two major groups of *sexual and gender identity disorders;* includes *sexual desire disorders, sexual arousal disorders, orgasm disorders, sexual pain disorders,* sexual dysfunction due to a *general medical condition,* and substance-induced (intoxication/withdrawal) sexual dysfunction.

sexual masochism See *masochism, sexual.*

sexual pain disorders One group of *sexual dysfunctions* that includes dyspareunia and vaginismus. Dyspareunia refers to genital pain, in either a male or a female, before, during, or after sexual intercourse that is not due to a *general medical condition,* drugs, or medication. Vaginismus refers to recurrent or persistent involuntary spasm of the musculature of the outer third of the vagina severe enough to interfere with coitus.

sexual sadism See *sadism, sexual.*

shaman A healer whose ability comes from trancelike or supernatural experiences.

shame An *emotion* resulting from the failure to live up to self-expectations. See also *guilt; superego.*

shaping Reinforcement of responses in the patient's repertoire that increasingly approximate sought-after behavior.

shell shock Term used in World War I to designate a wide variety of *mental disorders* presumably due to combat experience. See also *combat fatigue.*

shock treatment An inaccurate term often used to refer to *electroconvulsive therapy.*

short-term memory The recognition, recall, and reproduction of perceived material 10 seconds or longer after initial presentation. See also *immediate memory.*

sibling A full brother or sister.

sibling relational problem See *relational problems.*

sibling rivalry The competition between *siblings* for the love of a parent or for other recognition or gain.

sick role An identity adopted by an individual as a "patient" that specifies a set of expected behaviors, usually dependent.

side effect A drug response that accompanies the principal response for which a medication is taken. Most side effects are undesirable yet cause only minor annoyances; others may cause serious problems.

sign Objective evidence of disease or disorder. See also *symptom.*

signal anxiety An *ego* mechanism that results in activation of defensive operations to protect the ego from being overwhelmed by an excess of excitement. The *anxiety* reaction that was originally experienced in a traumatic situation is reproduced in an attenuated form, allowing defenses to be mobilized before the current threat does, in fact, become overwhelming.

simple phobia Specific *phobia.*

simple schizophrenia See *schizophrenia.*

Skinner, Burrhus Frederic (1904–1990) American *psychologist* noted for his research and writings on *operant conditioning.* Many of the procedures of *behavior therapy* are based on laboratory research by Skinner and his students.

sleep The recurring period of relative physical and psychological disengagement from one's environment accompanied by characteristic EEG (*electroencephalogram*) findings and divisible into two categories: non–rapid eye movement (NREM) sleep, also known as orthodox or synchronized (S) sleep; and rapid eye movement (REM) sleep, also referred to as paradoxical or desynchronized (D) sleep. Dreaming sleep is another, though less accurate, term for REM sleep. Four stages of NREM sleep based on EEG findings are stage 1, occurring immediately after sleep begins, with a pattern of low amplitude and fast frequency; stage 2, having characteristic waves of 12 to 16 cycles per second, known as sleep spindles; and stages 3 and 4, having progressive further slowing of frequency and increase in amplitude of the wave forms.

Over a period of 90 minutes after the beginning of sleep, a person has progressed through the four stages of NREM sleep and emerges from them into the first period of REM sleep. REM sleep is associated with dreaming, and brief cycles (20 to 30 minutes) of this sleep recur about every 90 minutes throughout the night. Coordinated rapid eye movements give this type of sleep its name. Sleep patterns vary with age, state of health, medication, and psychological state. See also *sleep disorders; sleep terror disorder; somnambulism.*

sleep apnea Temporarily not breathing while asleep. Its most common cause is obstruction of the airway by excessive tissue. See *breathing-related sleep disorder.*

sleep disorders In DSM-IV, this category includes primary sleep disorders (*dyssomnias* and *parasomnias*), sleep disorders (*insomnia* or *hypersomnia*) related to another *mental disorder,* secondary sleep disorder due to a *general medical condition,* and substance-induced (intoxication/withdrawal) sleep disorder.

sleep terror disorder One of the *parasomnias,* characterized by *panic* and confusion when abruptly awakening from *sleep.* This usually begins with a scream and is accompanied by intense *anxiety.* The person is often confused and disoriented after awakening. No detailed dream is recalled, and there is *amnesia* for the episode. Sleep terrors typically occur during the first third of the major sleep episode. Contrast with *nightmare disorder.*

sleep-wake schedule disorder See *circadian rhythm sleep disorder.*

sleepwalking disorder One of the *parasomnias,* characterized by recurrent episodes of arising from the bed during *sleep* and walking about. The sleepwalking person has a blank, staring face and is relatively unresponsive to attempts by others to awaken him or her. On awakening, either from the sleepwalking episode or the next morning, the person has *amnesia* for the episode. Sleepwalking typically occurs during the first third of the major sleep episode.

smooth pursuit eye movements (SPEM) A tracking system that enables the viewer to keep a moving target in focus. See *eye tracking.*

social adaptation The ability to live and express oneself according to society's restrictions and cultural demands.

social anthropology The study of human society, with emphasis on the development of institutions, social roles, tribal organization, community structure, political systems, economic organization, and so forth. See *cultural anthropology; ethnology.*

social breakdown syndrome The concept that some psychiatric symptomatology is a result of treatment conditions and inadequate facilities and not a part of the primary illness. Factors bringing about the condition are social labeling, learning the role of the chronically sick, atrophy of work and social skills, and *identification* with the sick. See also *rehabilitation.*

social phobia See *phobia.*

social psychiatry The field of *psychiatry* concerned with the cultural, ecological, and sociological factors that engender, precipitate, intensify, prolong, or otherwise complicate maladaptive patterns of behavior and their treatment.

social viscosity See *interictal behavior syndrome.*

social work A profession whose primary concern is how human needs—both of individuals and of groups—can be met within society. Social and behavioral sciences provide its educational base. Practice methods are directed to fostering maximal growth and development in people and to influencing their environments to become more responsive to their needs. The services provided include general social services, such as health and education, and welfare services to targeted groups such as the economically disadvantaged, the disabled, the elderly, or victims of disasters.

A social worker may focus on the individual in need and do casework; work with families, marital partnerships, groups of veterans, or prison inmates and do group work; or emphasize social change and community organization.

The medical social worker typically performs three overlapping functions: 1) assesses the social and psychological factors that have affected the development of an illness or are likely to be significant in the treatment and rehabilitation; 2) helps the patient and family to identify and use appropriately resources and facilities of all types; and 3) prepares the family and the community for the return of the patient and particular challenges that might be posed. See *clinical social worker; psychiatric social worker.*

socialization The process by which society integrates the person and the way he or she learns to become a functioning member of that society. See also *sociology.*

sociobiology The study of the evolution of social behavior. This field of study is rooted in evolutionary biology, *ethology,* and comparative *psychology.*

sociology The study of the governing principles and development of social organization and the group behavior of people, in contrast to individual behavior. It overlaps to some extent with anthropology. See also *alienation; socialization.*

sociometry The science of assessing the interpersonal psychological structure of a group or society.

sociopath An unofficial term for *antisocial personality.* See *personality disorder.*

sociotherapy Any treatment in which emphasis is on socioenvironmental and interpersonal rather than *intrapsychic* factors, as in the *therapeutic community.* In most forms of sociotherapy, peer acceptance is an important element, typically achieved through confrontation by the group when peer expectations are not met.

sodomy Anal intercourse. Legally, the term may include other types of perversion such as *bestiality.* See also *paraphilia.*

soma The body.

somatic delusion See *delusional disorder.*

somatic therapy In *psychiatry,* the biological treatment of mental disorders (e.g., *electroconvulsive therapy,* psychopharmacological treatment). Contrast with *psychotherapy.*

somatization disorder One of the *somatoform disorders,* characterized by multiple physical complaints not fully explained by any known medical condition yet severe enough to result in medical treatment or alteration in lifestyle. *Symptoms* include pain in different sites and other symptoms referable to the gastrointestinal tract and the sexual/reproductive system, or those suggestive of neurologic involvement.

somatoform disorders A group of disorders with *symptoms* suggesting physical disorders but without demonstrable organic findings to explain the symptoms. There is positive evidence, or a strong presumption, that the symptoms are linked to psychological factors or *conflicts*. In DSM-IV, this category includes *somatization disorder, conversion disorder, hypochondriasis, body dysmorphic disorder,* and *pain disorder*. Included as a somatoform disorder not otherwise specified is *pseudocyesis*.

specific phobia See *phobia*.

speech and language disorders See *communication disorders*.

speech disturbance Any disorder of verbal communication that is not due to faulty innervation of speech muscles or organs of articulation. The term includes many language and *learning disabilities*. Contrast with *agraphia, aphasia,* and *apraxia* in LIST OF NEUROLOGIC DEFICITS. See also *amimia; dyslexia*.

SPEM *Smooth pursuit eye movements*.

splitting A mental mechanism in which the self or others are reviewed as all good or all bad, with failure to integrate the positive and negative qualities of self and others into cohesive images. Often the person alternately idealizes and devalues the same person.

standard deviation See LIST OF RESEARCH TERMS.

Stanford-Binet Intelligence Scale See TABLE OF PSYCHOLOGICAL TESTS.

status epilepticus Continuous epileptic seizures. See *epilepsy*.

stepwise deterioration See *dementia, vascular*.

stereotypic movement disorder Stereotypy/habit disorder; a disorder of infancy, childhood, or adolescence characterized by repetitive, driven, nonfunctional, and potentially self-injurious behavior such as head banging, self-biting, or picking at the skin. The behavior may be associated with *mental retardation* or a *pervasive developmental disorder.*

steroids, anabolic Synthetic derivatives of testosterone used medically to promote protein anabolism. They can be drugs of abuse used to aid in body building. They sometimes produce an initial sense of well-being replaced after repeated use by lack of energy, irritability, and unhappiness. Continued use may lead to such serious complications as severe *depression,* outbursts of violence, and liver disease.

stimulants See TABLE OF DRUGS USED IN PSYCHIATRY.

Stockholm syndrome A kidnapping or terrorist hostage identifies with and has sympathy for his or her captors on whom he or she is dependent for survival.

street drugs See TABLE OF COMMONLY ABUSED DRUGS.

strephosymbolia A tendency to reverse letters and words in reading and writing. Seen in *learning disability.*

stress disorder, acute Brief reactive *dissociative disorder;* an *anxiety disorder* that develops while the person experiences (or immediately thereafter) actual or threatened injury or death, or witnesses the serious injury or killing of another person. The episode is short-lived (less than 4 weeks) but interferes with functioning, often preventing the person from taking appropriate action to obtain medical, legal, or family assistance. *Symptoms* may include any combination of the following: *stupor, derealization, depersonalization, amnesia,* a sense of numbing or detachment, feelings of fear or terror, palpitations, muscle tension, fatigue, intrusive recollections of the incident, sleep disturbance, anger, agitation, or feelings of hopelessness.

stress disorder/reaction, posttraumatic See *posttraumatic stress disorder.*

stress reaction An acute, maladaptive emotional response to industrial, domestic, civilian, or military disasters, and other calamitous life situations; it may also be chronic, as seen in some Vietnam veterans. See *posttraumatic stress disorder.*

stroke Cerebrovascular accident (CVA); *apoplexy;* gross cerebral hemorrhage or softening of the brain following hemorrhage, thrombosis, or embolism of the cerebral arteries. *Symptoms* may include *coma,* paralysis (particularly on one side of the body), *convulsions, aphasia,* and other neurologic signs determined by the location of the lesion.

structural integration See *experiential therapy.*

structural theory *Freud's* model of the mental apparatus composed of *id, ego,* and *superego.*

stupor Marked decrease in reactivity to and awareness of the environment, with reduced spontaneous movements and activity. It can be seen as a type of *catatonic behavior* in *schizophrenia,* but it can also be observed in neurologic disorders.

stuttering A *communication disorder* characterized by disturbance of the fluency and time patterning of speech; *symptoms* may include repetitions of sounds or syllables, sound prolongations, interjections, or circumlocutions to avoid difficult words.

subconscious Obsolete term. Formerly used to include the *preconscious* (what can be recalled with effort) and the *unconscious.*

sublimation A *defense mechanism,* operating unconsciously, by which instinctual *drives,* consciously unacceptable, are diverted into personally and socially acceptable channels.

substance A chemical agent that is used intentionally to alter mood or behavior (*psychoactive substance*). Also includes prescribed medications and poisons, toxins, industrial solvents, and other agents to which one may be exposed unintentionally and whose effects on the nervous system may lead to behavioral or cognitive disturbances.

substance abuse See *abuse, substance.*

Substance Abuse and Mental Health Services Administration (SAMHSA) An agency of the U.S. Department of Health and Human Services created in 1992 and made up of the Center for Mental Health Services, the Center for Substance Abuse Prevention, and the Center for Substance Abuse Treatment. These programs were formerly contained in the Alcohol, Drug Abuse, and Mental Health Administration.

substance, dependence See *dependence, substance.*

substance related disorders In DSM-IV, this category includes *substance use disorders* and *substance-induced mental disorders.*

substance use disorders *Dependence,* abuse, intoxication, and withdrawal syndromes associated with regular or episodic use of chemical substances. Use disorders are recognized for alcohol, amphetamine, caffeine, cannabis, cocaine, hallucinogen, inhalant, nicotine, opioid, phencyclidine, sedative/hypnotic/anxiolytic drugs, and for combinations of drugs (polysubstance).

Specific disorders include dependence (for all of the above mentioned substances except caffeine); abuse (for all except caffeine and nicotine); intoxication (for all except nicotine); and withdrawal (for all except caffeine, cannabis, hallucinogen, inhalant, and phencyclidine).

substance-induced mental disorders Mental syndromes secondary to the use of drugs (including alcohol). In DSM-IV, these disorders (except for intoxication and withdrawal) are placed in the diagnostic categories with which they share phenomenology. For example, substance-induced mood disorder is listed under mood disorders and substance-induced sleep disorder is listed under sleep disorders. See *organic.*

The classifications include *delirium, dementia, amnestic disorder, psychotic disorder* with delusions or hallucinations, *mood disorder, anxiety disorder, sleep disorder,* and *sexual dysfunction.*

Substance-induced mental disorders have a three-part name in DSM-IV: the name of the specific substance (alcohol, cocaine, etc.); an indication of whether it is intoxication, withdrawal, or persists beyond these times; and the specific presentation (mood disorder, anxiety disorder, etc.). Examples are alcohol persisting amnestic disorder or cocaine withdrawal mood disorder with depressive features.

substance-induced psychotic disorder This DSM-IV term combines the two disorders that in DSM-III-R were called psychoactive substance–induced delusional disorder and psychoactive substance–induced hallucinosis into a single category. The prominent features are *hallucinations* or *delusions* that develop during use of a substance or within 6 weeks of stopping its use. Such conditions have been described during alcohol *intoxication* and *withdrawal,* intoxication and withdrawal from *sedative/hypnotic/anxiolytic drugs,* and intoxication with *amphetamines, cannabis, cocaine, hallucinogens,* inhalants, *opioids,* and *phencyclidine.*

substitution A *defense mechanism,* operating unconsciously, by which an unattainable or unacceptable goal, *emotion,* or object is replaced by one that is more attainable or acceptable.

succinylcholine A short-acting anticholinesterase drug used intravenously in *anesthesia* as a skeletal muscle relaxant. Also used in conjunction with *elec-*

troconvulsive therapy to minimize the possibility of complications.

suggestibility Uncritical compliance or acceptance of an idea, belief, or attribute.

suggestion The process of influencing a patient to accept an idea, belief, or attitude suggested by the therapist. See also *hypnosis*.

suicide Taking of one's own life.

suicide, cluster See *cluster suicides*.

Sullivan, Harry Stack (1892–1949) American *psychiatrist* and *psychoanalyst* known for his research on the *psychotherapy* of *schizophrenia* and for his view of complex interpersonal relationships as the basis of *personality* development.

superego In psychoanalytic theory (see *psychoanalysis*), that part of the *personality* structure associated with ethics, standards, and self-criticism. It is formed by *identification* with important and esteemed persons in early life, particularly parents. The supposed or actual wishes of these significant persons are taken over as part of the child's own standards to help form the *conscience*. See also *ego; guilt; id; shame*.

supportive psychotherapy A type of therapy in which the therapist-patient relationship is used to help the patient cope with specific crises or difficulties that he or she is currently facing. Supportive therapy avoids, rather than encourages, the development of *transference* neurosis. It employs a range of techniques, depending on the patient's strengths and weaknesses and the particular problems that are currently distressing. These techniques include listening in a sympathetic, concerned, understanding, and non-judgmental fashion; providing factual information that may counter a patient's unrealistic fears; setting limits and encouraging the patient to control or relinquish self-destructive behavior and to give attention to more constructive action; and facilitating discharge of and relief from painful feelings within the controlled environment of the consultation room. See also *psychotherapy.*

suppression The *conscious* effort to control and conceal unacceptable impulses, thoughts, feelings, or acts.

symbiosis A mutually reinforcing relationship between two persons who are dependent on each other; a normal characteristic of the relationship between the mother and infant child. See *separation-individuation.*

symbiotic psychosis A condition seen in 2- to 4-year-old children with an abnormal relationship to a mothering figure. The *psychosis* is characterized by intense *separation anxiety,* severe *regression,* giving up of useful speech, and *autism.* See *exogenous psychoses.*

symbolization A general mechanism in all human thinking by which some mental representation comes to stand for some other thing, class of things, or attribute of something. This mechanism underlies dream formation and some *symptoms,* such as conversion reactions, *obsessions,* and *compulsions.* The link between the latent meaning of the symptom and the symbol is usually *unconscious.*

sympathetic nervous system The part of the *autonomic nervous system* that responds to dangerous or threatening situations by preparing a person physiologically for "fight or flight." See also *parasympathetic nervous system.*

sympathy A feeling or capacity for sharing in the interests or concerns of another. May arise when there is no emotional attachment to the person toward whom one is sympathetic because the feelings of the sympathetic person remain essentially internal. Contrast with *empathy.*

symptom A specific manifestation of a patient's condition indicative of an abnormal physical or mental state; a subjective perception of illness.

symptomatic psychoses See *organic mental disorder.*

synapse The gap between the membrane of one nerve cell and the membrane of another. The synapse is the space through which the nerve impulse is passed, chemically or electrically, from one nerve to another.

syndrome A configuration of *symptoms* that occur together and constitute a recognizable condition.

syntaxic mode The mode of perception that forms whole, logical, coherent pictures of reality that can be validated by others.

syphilis A sexually transmitted venereal disease, which, if untreated, may lead to *central nervous system* deterioration with psychotic manifestations in its later stages. See also *general paralysis.*

systematic desensitization A *behavior therapy* procedure widely used to modify behaviors associated with *phobias.* The procedure involves the construction of a hierarchy of *anxiety*-producing stimuli by the subject, and gradual presentation of the stimuli until they no longer produce anxiety. Also called desensitization. See also *reciprocal inhibition.*

T

taboo Prohibition or restriction interwoven in the culture.

talion law or principle A primitive, unrealistic belief, usually *unconscious,* conforming to the Biblical injunction of "an eye for an eye and a tooth for a tooth." In *psychoanalysis,* the concept and fear that all injury, actual or intended, will be punished in kind.

tangentiality Replying to a question in an oblique or irrelevant way. Compare with *circumstantiality.*

tangle, neurofibrillary See *Alzheimer's disease.*

Tarasoff decision A California court decision that essentially imposes a duty on the therapist to warn the appropriate person or persons when the therapist becomes aware that the patient may present a risk of harm to a specific person or persons. See also LIST OF LEGAL TERMS.

tardive dyskinesia, neuroleptic-induced A medication-induced movement disorder consisting of involuntary choreiform, athetoid, or rhythmic movements of the tongue, jaw, or extremities developing with long-term use (usually a few months or more) of neuroleptic medication.

TAT (Thematic Apperception Test) See TABLE OF PSYCHOLOGICAL TESTS.

telepathy Communication of thought from one person to another without the intervention of physical means. See also *extrasensory perception; parapsychology.*

telephone scatologia One of the *paraphilias,* characterized by marked distress over, or acting on, sexual urges that involve telephone calls to a nonconsenting listener in order to verbalize erotic or obscene language (lewdness).

temperament Constitutional predisposition to react in a particular way to stimuli.

temporal lobe One of the four major subdivisions of each hemisphere of the cerebral cortex of the brain. It functions in speech and in auditory and complex visual perceptions.

temporal lobe epilepsy Complex partial seizures; psychomotor epilepsy. See *epilepsy.*

temporal lobe syndromes Mental and behavior disturbances associated with *temporal lobe epilepsy* or other temporal lobe pathology. Lesions in the dominant temporal lobe may produce auditory *hallucinations,* primary *delusions, formal thought disorder,* and impaired verbal and reading comprehension. Lesions in the nondominant temporal lobe may produce *depression,* inappropriate emotional expression, and impaired visual and auditory memory.

termination The act of ending or concluding. In *psychotherapy,* termination refers to the mutual agreement between patient and therapist to bring therapy to an end. The idea of termination often occurs to both, but usually it is the therapist who introduces the subject into the session as a possibility to be considered. In *psychoanalytic* treatment (see *psychoanalysis*), the patient's reactions are worked through to completion before the treatment ends. The early termination that is characteristic of focal psychotherapy and other forms of *brief psychotherapy* often requires more extensive work with the feelings of loss and separation.

tertiary prevention See *prevention.*

testamentary capacity See LIST OF LEGAL TERMS.

thalamus Consists of two egg-shaped masses of nerve tissue deep within the brain. It is an important relay station, which seems to act as a filter, for sensory information flowing into the brain. The thalamus also may play a part in *short-* and *long-term memory.*

thanatology The study of death and dying, emphasizing therapeutic interventions with dying persons and their survivors.

therapeutic community A term of British origin, now widely used, for a specially structured mental hospital milieu that encourages patients to function within the range of social norms.

therapeutic window A well-defined range of *blood levels* associated with optimal clinical response to antidepressant drugs, such as nortriptyline. Levels above or below that range are associated with a poor response.

thioxanthene derivatives See TABLE OF DRUGS USED IN PSYCHIATRY.

third ear (the) Utilization of intuition, sensitivity, and awareness of subliminal cues to interpret clinical observations of patients in therapy.

third-party payer Any organization (public or private) that pays or insures health or medical expenses on behalf of beneficiaries or recipients. Examples are *Medicare, Medicaid,* and Blue Cross and Blue Shield and other commercial insurance companies.

thought disorder A disturbance of speech, communication, or content of thought, such as *delusions, ideas of reference,* poverty of thought, *flight of ideas, perseveration, loosening of associations,* and so forth. A thought disorder can be caused by a functional emotional disorder or an organic condition. A formal thought disorder is a disturbance in the form of thought rather than in the content of thought (e.g., loosening of associations).

tic An involuntary, sudden, rapid, recurrent, nonrhythmic stereotyped motor movement or vocalization. A tic may be an expression of an emotional conflict, the result of *neurologic* disease, or an effect of a drug (especially a stimulant or other *dopamine agonist*).

tic disorders In DSM-IV, this category includes *Tourette's disorder,* chronic motor or vocal tic disorder, transient tic disorder, and tic disorder not otherwise specified; all beginning before the age of 18 years. Chronic tics may occur many times a day, nearly every day, or intermittently over a period of more than a year. Transient tics do not persist for longer than 12 consecutive months.

TM Transcendental meditation. See *experiential therapy.*

token economy A system involving the application of the principles and procedures of *operant conditioning* to the management of a social setting such as a ward, classroom, or halfway house. Tokens are given contingent on completion of specified activities and are exchangeable for goods or privileges desired by the patient.

tolerance A characteristic of substance dependence that may be shown by the need for markedly increased amounts of the substance to achieve intoxication or the desired effect, by markedly diminished effect with continued use of the same amount of the substance, or by adequate functioning despite doses or blood levels of the substance that would be expected to produce significant impairment in a casual user.

tomography Radiologic imaging of serial planes ("cuts") through an anatomic structure. See also *brain imaging.*

topographic model *Freud's* model of the structure of the mind, first described in terms of the *conscious-preconscious-unconscious* and a simple conflict theory of the conscious opposing the unconscious. This model was replaced later by the more complex model of *id, ego,* and *superego,* and its correlated concept of intersystemic conflicts. This led to a shift in clinical focus from discovery of unconscious drive-related wishes to systematic analysis of the ego's unconscious defensive operations.

toucherism See *frotteurism.*

Tourette's disorder A *tic disorder* consisting of multiple motor and vocal tics that occur in bouts, either concurrently or separately, almost every day or intermittently over a period of more than 12 months.

toxic psychosis An *organic mental disorder* caused by the poisonous effect of chemicals or drugs.

toxicity The capacity of a drug to damage body tissue or seriously impair body functions.

trance A state of focused attention and diminished sensory and motor activity seen in *hypnosis; hysterical neurosis, dissociative type* (see under *neurosis*); and ecstatic religious states.

trance disorder, dissociative Of the *dissociative disorders,* the one most frequently reported in non-Western cultures, characterized by a disturbance of the normally integrative functions of *memory, identity,* or consciousness, or by a conviction of having been taken over by a spirit, deity, or other person (i.e., possession). In a *trance,* consciousness is altered and responsivity is markedly diminished or selectively focused. Other dissociative phenomena may include amnestic episodes and the assumption of a different identity. The *symptoms* cause great distress or significant impairment in functioning, and they fall outside the sanctioned religious practices of the community.

Many different *culture-specific syndromes,* indigenous to particular locations and cultures and predominated by trance and possession phenomena, have been described. See *culture-specific syndromes.*

tranquilizer A drug that decreases *anxiety* and *agitation.* Preferred terms are antianxiety and antipsychotic drugs. See also TABLE OF DRUGS USED IN PSYCHIATRY.

transactional analysis A psychodynamic *psychotherapy* based on role theory that attempts to understand the interplay between therapist and patient and ultimately between the patient and external reality. See also OUTLINE OF SCHOOLS OF PSYCHIATRY.

transcendental meditation See *experiential therapy.*

transcultural psychiatry See *cross-cultural psychiatry.*

transference The *unconscious* assignment to others of feelings and attitudes that were originally associated with important figures (parents, *siblings,* etc.) in one's early life. The transference relationship follows the pattern of its prototype. The *psychiatrist* utilizes this phenomenon as a therapeutic tool to help the patient understand emotional problems and their origins. In the patient-physician relationship, the transference

may be negative (hostile) or positive (affectionate).
See also *countertransference; parataxic distortion.*

transference cure Flight into health; the patient flees
from further treatment in order to avoid dealing with
repressed material. The *neurosis* is not cured but is in
temporary *remission;* relapses are almost certain when
the patient encounters further stress.

transference, selfobject In the *self psychology* of
Kohut, a *transference* relationship in which the therapist serves as a *selfobject* for the patient by providing
needed self-enhancing and self-regulatory functions
and emotional stability, which can subsequently be
internalized and transformed into the structure of the
patient's self. The therapist functions as a needed
extension of the patient's self rather than as a separate
person. Three major types of selfobject transference
are recognized: *mirroring,* idealizing, and alter-ego
(twinship).

transient tic disorder See *tic disorders.*

transitional object An object, other than the mother,
selected by an infant between 4 and 18 months of age
for self-soothing and *anxiety*-reduction. Examples are
a "security blanket" or a toy that helps the infant go
to sleep. The transitional object provides an opportunity to master external objects and promotes the
differentiation of self from outer world.

transsexualism See *gender identity disorder.*

transvestism Sexual pleasure derived from dressing or
masquerading in the clothing of the opposite sex, with
the strong wish to appear as a member of the opposite
sex. The sexual origins of transvestism may be *unconscious.*

trauma, psychic An *intrapsychic* event brought on by
exposure to an anticipated danger. The acute *syndrome* is characterized by psychological shock; helplessness; numbness of feelings; disturbances of
speech, eating, and sleeping (nightmares); and social

withdrawal. Persistence of the helpless state may result in death. The long-term effects are usually persistent narcissistic preoccupation; *somatic* concerns; depressive and *anxiety* symptoms; and fear of being further victimized. See *posttraumatic stress disorder.*

traumatic neurosis See *posttraumatic stress disorder.*

treatment resistance Lack of response to a specific therapy that would ordinarily be expected to be effective. The patient who does not respond to the usual dosage of a drug but does respond to a higher dosage is often termed a "relative resister." Absolute resistance refers to the patient who fails to respond to any dosage of the drug.

tremor A trembling or shaking of the body or any of its parts. It may be induced by medication.

trichotillomania Pathological hair pulling that results in noticeable hair loss. As in other *impulse control disorders,* an increasing sense of tension or affective arousal immediately precedes an episode of hair pulling, which is then followed by a sense of pleasure, gratification, or relief.

tricyclic antidepressants See TABLE OF DRUGS USED IN PSYCHIATRY.

trisomy The presence of three *chromosomes* instead of the two that normally represent each potential set of chromosomes. This can result in a developmental disability. An example of trisomy is *Down syndrome.*

Tuke, William (1732–1822) English Quaker who pioneered the treatment of psychiatric patients without using physical restraints.

Turner syndrome A *chromosomal* defect in women with a karyotype of XO and 45 chromosomes rather than the usual 46. Clinical features of this disorder are small stature, webbed neck, abnormal ovarian development, and sometimes *mental retardation.*

twin research A powerful method of investigating the relative degree of phenotypic variance that can be attributed to genetic factors and to transmissible and nontransmissible environmental factors. For example, the dissimilarities between *monozygotic* twins are compared with the behavioral variations occurring in nontwin siblings or *dizygotic twins.*

twinship transference See *transference, selfobject.*

type A personality A *temperament* characterized by excessive drive, competitiveness, a sense of time urgency, impatience, unrealistic ambition, and need for control. Believed to be associated with a high incidence of coronary artery disease.

type B personality A *temperament* characterized by a relaxed, easy-going demeanor; less time-bound and competitive than the *type A personality.*

tyramine A sympathomimetic *amine* that acts by displacing stored transmitter from adrenergic axonal terminals; a constituent of many foods such as flat beans, cheese, red wine, and so forth, which are forbidden when using *monoamine oxidase inhibitors* because of *hypertensive crisis.*

U

ultradian rhythms See *biological rhythms.*

unconscious That part of the mind or mental functioning of which the content is only rarely subject to awareness. It is a repository for data that have never been *conscious* (primary *repression*) or that may have been conscious and are later repressed (secondary repression).

undifferentiated schizophrenia See *schizophrenia.*

undoing A mental mechanism consisting of behavior that symbolically atones for, makes amends for, or reverses previous thoughts, feelings, or actions.

unipolar psychoses Recurrent major depressions. See *depression*.

urophilia One of the *paraphilias,* characterized by marked distress over, or acting on, sexual urges that involve urine.

use disorders See *substance use disorders*.

utilization review committee A committee of physicians and other clinical staff formed in a hospital to review the quality of services rendered, as well as the effective and appropriate use of facilities. See also *peer review organization*.

V

---

vaginismus See *sexual pain disorders*.

variance See LIST OF RESEARCH TERMS.

vascular dementia See *dementia, vascular*.

vegetative nervous system Obsolete term for *autonomic nervous system*.

verbigeration Stereotyped and seemingly meaningless repetition of words or sentences. See also *perseveration*.

vertigo A sensation that the external world is spinning around; a *symptom* of vestibular dysfunction.

viscosity, social See *interictal behavior syndrome*.

vitamin therapy See *orthomolecular treatment*.

vocal tic disorder See *tic disorders*.

voice disorder A *communication disorder* characterized by abnormal vocal pitch, loudness, quality, tone, or resonance of enough severity to interfere with educational or occupational achievement or with social communication. Unlike other communication disorders, voice disorder may not appear until adulthood.

voluntary admission See *commitment*.

voyeurism Peeping; one of the *paraphilias,* characterized by marked distress over, or acting on, urges to
observe unsuspecting people, usually strangers, who
are naked or in the process of disrobing, or who are
engaging in sexual activity.

W

Wagner von Jauregg, Julius (1857–1940) Austrian
neuropsychiatrist who won the Nobel Prize in 1927
for research in using malaria inoculation and other
artificially induced fevers in treating syphilis of the
central nervous system.

watchfulness, frozen See *attachment disorder, reactive; frozen watchfulness.*

Watson, John B. (1878–1958) American *psychologist*
and founder of the behaviorism school of *psychology.*

waxy flexibility See *cerea flexibilitas; schizophrenia.*

Wechsler Adult Intelligence Scale (WAIS) See TABLE
OF PSYCHOLOGICAL TESTS.

weekend hospitalization See *partial hospitalization.*

Wernicke-Korsakoff syndrome A disease of *central
nervous system* metabolism due to a lack of vitamin
B_1 (thiamine) seen in chronic *alcoholism.* Wernicke's
disease features irregularities of eye movements, incoordination, impaired thinking, and often sensorimotor
deficits. *Korsakoff's syndrome* is characterized by *confabulation* and, more importantly, by a short-term, but
not immediate, disturbance that leads to gross impairment in memory and learning. Wernicke's disease and
Korsakoff's psychosis begin suddenly and are often
found in the same person simultaneously. See also
alcohol psychosis.

Weyer, Johann (circa 1530) Dutch physician who was one of the first to devote his major interest to psychiatric disorders. Regarded by some as the founder of modern *psychiatry,* he viewed the phenomena of witchcraft as *symptoms* of *mental illness* and strongly opposed the religious persecution of those accused of practicing witchcraft.

White, William Alanson (1870–1937) American *psychiatrist* famous for his early support of *psychoanalysis* and his contributions to *forensic psychiatry.*

windigo See *culture-specific syndromes.*

withdrawal A pathological retreat from people or the world of reality, often seen in *schizophrenia.*

withdrawal symptoms The constellation of *symptoms* and signs that develops within a short period of time (usually hours) after cessation or significant reduction of use of a substance in a person with a pattern of heavy or prolonged use of the substance. The withdrawal syndrome tends to be specific for each substance.

> **alcohol** Within hours of cessation of, or significant reduction in, alcohol use in a person with a pattern of heavy and prolonged drinking, the subject develops hand *tremor* and a variety of associated *symptoms* that may include nausea and vomiting; *anxiety;* perceptual disturbances such as transient visual, tactile, or auditory *hallucinations* or *illusions* with intact *reality testing;* sweating or increased pulse rate; *psychomotor agitation; insomnia;* and grand mal seizures. The most severe form is *delirium tremens.* See *delirium.*
>
> **amphetamine** Cessation of prolonged heavy use of amphetamine or related substance produces a *dysphoric* mood and physiological changes such as fatigue, vivid and unpleasant dreams, *insomnia* or *hypersomnia,* and increased appetite.

cocaine *Symptoms* and signs are the same as in amphetamine withdrawal (see above).

nicotine Abrupt cessation of, or reduction in, nicotine use induces any combination of the following: dysphoric or depressed mood, *insomnia,* irritability or anger, *anxiety,* difficulty in concentrating, restlessness, decreased heart rate, and increased appetite or weight gain.

opioid The syndrome follows cessation of prolonged moderate or heavy use of an opioid, or reduction in the amount of opioid used, or administration of an opioid *antagonist. Symptoms* include dysphoric mood, nausea or vomiting, muscle aches, lacrimation or *rhinorrhea,* pupillary dilation, *piloerection,* sweating, diarrhea, yawning, fever, and *insomnia.*

sedative/hypnotic/anxiolytic Symptoms and signs are the same as described for alcohol withdrawal (see above).

word salad A mixture of words and phrases that lack comprehensive meaning or logical coherence; commonly seen in schizophrenic states (see *schizophrenia*).

word-blindness See *learning disability.*

working through Exploration of a problem by patient and therapist until a satisfactory solution has been found or until a *symptom* has been traced to its *unconscious* sources.

World Psychiatric Association (WPA) A nongovernmental organization composed of about 75 member societies from as many countries. Its headquarters are based in the home country of its secretariat.

written expression, disorder of Developmental expressive writing disorder; an *academic skills disorder* characterized by a significantly lower than expected level of writing skills given the subject's age, intelligence, and age-appropriate education.

X

X-linkage Mode of genetic transmission in which a trait or *gene* is linked to the X chromosome. Has been implicated in some cases of *bipolar disorder*.

xenophobia See under *phobia*.

Y

yoga See *experiential therapy*.

Z

zeitgeist The general intellectual and cultural climate of taste characteristic of an era.

zoophilia One of the *paraphilias,* characterized by marked distress over, or acting on, urges to indulge in sexual activity that involves animals.

zygosity (dizygotic and monozygotic) See LIST OF RESEARCH TERMS.

References

American Psychiatric Association: Diagnostic and Statistical Manual of Mental Disorders, 3rd Edition, Revised. Washington, DC, American Psychiatric Association, 1987

American Psychiatric Association: Diagnostic and Statistical Manual of Mental Disorders, 4th Edition. Washington, DC, American Psychiatric Association, 1994

Campbell RJ: Psychiatric Dictionary, 6th Edition. New York, Oxford University Press, 1989

List of Commonly Used Abbreviations

AA Alcoholics Anonymous

AAAS American Association for the Advancement of Science

AABA American Anorexia/Bulimia Association

AACAP American Academy of Child and Adolescent Psychiatry

AACDP American Association of Chairmen of Departments of Psychiatry

AACP American Academy of Clinical Psychiatrists

AACP American Academy for Child Psychoanalysts

AACP American Association of Community Psychiatrists

AADPRT American Association of Directors of Psychiatric Residency Training

AAFP American Academy of Family Physicians

AAGP American Association for Geriatric Psychiatry

AAGHP American Association of General Hospital Psychiatrists

AAMC Association of American Medical Colleges

AAMD American Association on Mental Deficiency

AAMFT American Association for Marriage and Family Therapy

AAMR American Academy on Mental Retardation

AAN American Academy of Neurology

AANP American Association of Neuropathologists

AAP American Academy of Psychoanalysis

AAP American Academy of Psychotherapists

AAP Association for Academic Psychiatry

AAP Association for Advancement of Psychoanalysis

AAP Association for the Advancement of Psychotherapy

AAPA American Association of Psychiatric Administrators

AAPAA American Association of Psychiatrists in Alcoholism and Addictions

AAPC American Association of Pastoral Counselors

AAPH American Association for Partial Hospitalization

AAPL American Academy of Psychiatry and the Law

AAPSC American Association of Psychiatric Services for Children

AAPT Association for the Advancement of Psychotherapy

AAS American Association of Suicidology

AASP American Association for Social Psychiatry

AATA American Art Therapy Association

ABFP American Board of Forensic Psychiatry

ABMS American Board of Medical Specialties

ABPN American Board of Psychiatry and Neurology

ACMHA American College of Mental Health Administration

ACMPD American Council on Marijuana and Other Psychoactive Drugs

ACNP American College of Neuropsychiatrists

ACNPP American College of Neuropsychopharmacology

ACP American College of Physicians

ACP American College of Psychiatrists

ACP Association for Child Psychoanalysis

ACPA American College of Psychoanalysts

ACTH Adrenocorticotropic hormone

AD Alzheimer's disease

ADD attention-deficit disorder

ADHD attention-deficit/hyperactivity disorder (DSM-IV)

ADMSEP Association of Directors of Medical Student Education in Psychiatry

ADPANA Alcohol and Drug Problems Association of North America

ADRDA Alzheimer's Disease and Related Disorders Association

AFCR American Federation for Clinical Research

AFTA American Family Therapy Association

AGPA American Group Psychotherapy Association

AGS American Geriatrics Society

AHA American Hospital Association

AHCA American Health Care Association

AIBS American Institute of Biological Sciences

AIDS acquired immune deficiency syndrome

AIPP American Institute for Psychotherapy and Psycho-analysis

AIS American Institute of Stress

AJP *American Journal of Psychiatry*

AMA against medical advice

AMA American Medical Association

AMERSA Association of Medical Education and Research in Substance Abuse

AMHA Association of Mental Health Administrators

AMHC Association of Mental Health Clergy

AMHCA American Mental Health Counselors Association

AMHF American Mental Health Foundation

AMHF American Mental Health Fund

AMHL Association of Mental Health Librarians

AMSA American Medical Society on Alcoholism and Other Drug Dependencies

AMSA American Medical Student Association

AMWA American Medical Women's Association

ANA American Neurological Association

ANA American Nurses' Association

ANAD Anorexia Nervosa and Assorted Disorders (see NANAD)

ANFMP Association of Nervous and Former Mental Patients (Recovery, Inc.)

ANS autonomlc nervous system

AOA American Orthopsychiatric Association

AOTA American Occupational Therapy Association
APA American Psychiatric Association
APA American Psychoanalytic Association
APA American Psychological Association
APAL Asociacion Psiquitrica de America Latina
APM Academy of Psychosomatic Medicine
APPA American Psychopathological Association
APPI American Psychiatric Press, Inc.
APPM Association for Psychoanalytic and
  Psychosomatic Medicine
APS American Psychosomatic Society
ARC Association for Retarded Citizens of the U.S.
ARNMD Association for Research in Nervous and
  Mental Disease
ASA American Schizophrenia Association
ASAP American Society for Adolescent Psychiatry
ASF American Schizophrenia Foundation
ASGPP American Society of Group Psychotherapy and
  Psychodrama
ASLM American Society of Law and Medicine
ASPP American Society of Psychoanalytic Physicians
AWA away without authorization
BASH Bulimia Anorexia Self-Help, Inc.
BEAM brain electrical activity mapping
bid twice a day
BIS Brain Information Service
BMA British Medical Association
BRF Brain Research Foundation
BTRS Behavior Therapy and Research Society
CA Cocaine Anonymous
CARPA Caribbean Psychiatric Association
CAT Children's Apperception Test (see TABLE OF
  PSYCHOLOGICAL TESTS)
CAT computerized axial tomography
CBT cognitive-behavior therapy
CMA Canadian Medical Association
CME continuing medical education

CMHA Canadian Mental Health Association
CMHC community mental health center
CMSS Council of Medical Specialty Societies
CNS central nervous system
CPA Canadian Psychiatric Association
CPDD Committee on Problems of Drug Dependence
CPT Current Procedural Terminology (AMA)
CRF corticotropin-releasing factor
CSF cerebrospinal fluid
CT computed tomography
CVA cerebrovascular accident; stroke
CWLA Child Welfare League of America
DBH dopamine beta-hydroxylase
DHHS Department of Health and Human Services
DMH Department of Mental Health/Department of Mental Hygiene
DNA deoxyribonucleic acid
DOV discharged on visit
DRG diagnostic related group
DSM *Diagnostic and Statistical Manual of Mental Disorders*
DSM-IV *Diagnostic and Statistical Manual of Mental Disorders,* 4th Edition
DST Dexamethasone suppression test
DTs delirium tremens
ECA epidemiologic catchment area
ECFMG Educational Commission for Foreign Medical Graduates
ECT electroconvulsive therapy
EE expressed emotion
EEG electroencephalogram
EFA Epilepsy Foundation of America
EKG electrocardiogram; also ECG
EMG electromyogram
EPRA Eastern Psychiatric Research Association
ESP extrasensory perception
EST electroshock treatment

FDA Food and Drug Administration
FDMD Foundation for Depression and Manic Depression
GA Gamblers Anonymous
GAP Group for the Advancement of Psychiatry
GSR galvanic skin response
H&CP *Hospital and Community Psychiatry* (APA)
HIBR Huxley Institute for Biosocial Research
HMO health maintenance organization
HRSD Hamilton Rating Scale for Depression
HLTV-III virus involved in AIDS
IACPO Inter-American Council of Psychiatric Organizations
IALMH International Academy of Law and Mental Health
IASP International Association for Suicide Prevention
IASSMD International Association for the Scientific Study of Mental Deficiency
ICAMI International Committee Against Mental Illness
ICD *International Classification of Diseases*
ICSW International Council on Social Welfare
IFMP International Federation for Medical Psychotherapy
IFPS International Federation of Psychoanalytic Societies
IM/NAS Institute of Medicine/National Academy of Sciences
IND investigational new drug
IPT interpersonal psychotherapy
IQ intelligence quotient
ITAA International Transactional Analysis Association
JCAH Joint Commission on Accreditation of Hospitals (now JCAHO)
JCAHO Joint Commission on Accreditation of Healthcare Organizations
JCMHC Joint Commission on Mental Health of Children
JCMIH Joint Commission on Mental Illness and Health

JCPA Joint Commission on Public Affairs (APA)

LP lumbar puncture

LSD lysergic acid diethylamide

MAOI monoamine oxidase inhibitor

MBD minimal brain dysfunction

MDI manic-depressive illness

MHA Mental Health Association

MMPI Minnesota Multiphasic Personality Inventory (see TABLE OF PSYCHOLOGICAL TESTS)

MRAA Mental Retardation Association of America

MRI magnetic resonance imaging

NA Narcotics Anonymous

NADS National Association for Down Syndrome

NAIL Neurotics Anonymous International Liaison

NAMH National Association for Mental Health

NAMI National Alliance for the Mentally Ill

NAMT National Association for Music Therapy

NANAD National Association of Anorexia Nervosa and Associated Disorders (formerly Anorexia Nervosa and Associated Disorders)

NAPPH National Association of Private Psychiatric Hospitals (now NAPHS)

NARC National Association for Retarded Citizens

NARSD National Alliance for Research on Schizophrenia and Depression

NASMHPD National Association of State Mental Health Program Directors

NASW National Association of Social Workers

NAVACP National Association of Veterans Affairs Chiefs of Psychiatry

NBME National Board of Medical Examiners

NCA National Council on the Aging

NCADD National Council on Alcoholism and Drug Dependence

NCAI National Council on Alcoholism

NCCMHC National Council of Community Mental Health Centers

NCD National Council on Drugs

NDMDA National Depressive and Manic Depressive Association

NGCP National Guild of Catholic Psychiatrists

NHC National Health Council

NIA National Institute on Aging

NIAAA National Institute on Alcohol Abuse and Alcoholism

NIDA National Institute on Drug Abuse

NIMH National Institute of Mental Health

NLN National League for Nursing

NMA National Medical Association

NMHA National Mental Health Association

NMHF National Mental Health Foundation

NMS neuroleptic malignant syndrome

NOMIC National Organization for Mentally Ill Children

NRA National Rehabilitation Association

NRC National Research Council

NREM non–rapid eye movement (see *sleep*)

NSAC National Society for Autistic Children

NSF National Science Foundation

OBD organic brain disease

OBS organic brain syndrome

OCD obsessive-compulsive disorder

PCMH Public Committee on Mental Health

PDR *Physicians' Desk Reference*

PET positron-emission tomography

PKU phenylketonuria

PPA Philippine Psychiatrists of America

PSR Physicians for Social Responsibility

PSRO professional standards review organization

qid four times a day

RANZCP Royal Australian and New Zealand College of Psychiatrists

REM rapid eye movement (see *sleep*)

RCP Royal College of Psychiatrists

RCPSC Royal College of Physicians and Surgeons of Canada

RNA ribonucleic acid

RSM Royal Society of Medicine

SA Schizophrenics Anonymous

SAI Schizophrenics Anonymous International

SAD seasonal affective disorder

SAMHSA Substance Abuse and Mental Health Services Administration

SBM Society of Behavioral Medicine

SBP Society of Biological Psychiatry

SDAT senile dementia, Alzheimer type

SIECUS Sex Information and Education Council of the U.S.

SNS Society for Neuroscience

SPCP Society of Professors of Child Psychiatry

SMA Southern Medical Association

SPA Southern Psychiatric Association

SRS Sleep Research Society

SSI/SSDI Social Security Insurance/Social Security Disability Insurance

TIA transient ischemic attack

tid three times a day

TM transcendental meditation

TRH thyrotropin-releasing hormone

USPHS U.S. Public Health Service

VA Veterans Administration

WASP World Association for Social Psychiatry

WFMH World Federation for Mental Health

WHO World Health Organization

WMA World Medical Association

WPA World Psychiatric Association

WRAPD World Rehabilitation Association for the Psycho-Socially Disabled

Table of Drugs Used in Psychiatry

Generic name	Trade name(s) (examples)
ANTIANXIETY DRUGS	
Antihistamines	
diphenhydramine	Benadryl
hydroxyzine	Atarax, Vistaril
Benzodiazepines	
alprazolam	Xanax
chlordiazepoxide	Librium (and others)
clonazepam	Klonopin
clorazepate	Tranxene
diazepam	Valium
halazepam	Paxipam
lorazepam	Ativan
oxazepam	Serax
prazepam	Centrax
Azaspirodione	
buspirone hydrochloride	BuSpar
ANTIDEPRESSANT DRUGS	
Monoamine oxidase inhibitors	
isocarboxazid	Marplan
phenelzine	Nardil
selegiline, L-deprenyl	Eldepryl
tranylcypromine sulfate	Parnate

Tricyclics and similar compounds

amitriptyline	Amitril, Elavil, Endep
amoxapine	Asendin
clomipramine	Anafranil
desipramine	Norpramin, Pertofrane
doxepin	Adapin, Sinequan
imipramine	Tofranil (and others)
maprotiline	Ludiomil
nortriptyline	Aventyl, Pamelor
protriptyline	Vivactil
trimipramine	Surmontil

Serotonin reuptake inhibitors

clomipramine	Anafranil
fluoxetine	Prozac
paroxetine	Paxil
sertraline	Zoloft

Other agents

bupropion	Wellbutrin
trazodone	Desyrel

HYPNOTICS

Sedative-hypnotic* benzodiazepines

estazolam	Prosom
flurazepam	Dalmane
quazepam	Doral
temazepam	Restoril
triazolam	Halcion

ANTIMANIC DRUGS

lithium salts	
lithium carbonate	Eskalith, Lithane, Lithobid, Lithonate, Lithotabs
lithium citrate	Cibalith-S

---

*For examples of other sedative-hypnotic agents, see TABLE OF COMMONLY ABUSED DRUGS.

ANTICONVULSANTS

carbamazepine	Tegretol
valproic acid	Depakene, Depakote

ANTIPSYCHOTIC DRUGS

Butyrophenones

droperidol	Inapsine
haloperidol	Haldol

Dibenzazepines

clozapine	Clozaril
loxapine	Daxolin, Loxitane

Dihydroindolone

molindone	Lidone, Moban

Diphenylbutylpiperidine

pimozide	Orap

Phenothiazines

Aliphatic

chlorpromazine	Thorazine
triflupromazine	Vesprin

Piperazine

acetophenazine	Tindal
butaperazine	Repoise
carphenazine	Proketazine
fluphenazine	Prolixin, Permitil
perphenazine	Trilafon
trifluoperazine	Stelazine

Piperidine

mesoridazine	Serentil
piperacetazine	Quide
thioridazine	Mellaril

Thioxanthenes

chlorprothixene	Taractan
thiothixene	Navane

Table of Commonly Abused Drugs

Class	Trade name(s)	Street name(s)
Opioids		
morphine	morphine sulfate	dope, M, Miss Emma, morpho
heroin	none	H, junk, skag, boy, smack, horse
hydromorphone	Dilaudid	DL's
oxymorphone	Numorphan	
oxycodone	Percodan, Percocet	blues
meperidine	Demerol	Percs
methadone hydrochloride	Dolophine	dollys, done
pentazocine	Talwin	
tincture of opium	paregoric	PG, licorice
cough preparations with codeine	Elixir terpin hydrate, Robitussin A-C	schoolboy, blue velvet
hydrocodone	Hycodan	Robby
Non-narcotic analgesics		
propoxyphene	Darvon	

Class	Trade name(s)	Street name(s)
Benzodiazepines		**bennies, benzos**
diazepam	Valium	
chlordiazepoxide	Librium	
alprazolam	Xanax	
oxazepam	Serax	
lorazepam	Ativan	
Barbiturates		**barbs, candy, dolls, goofers, sleeping pills**
secobarbital sodium	Seconal	pink lady, red devils
amobarbital	Amytal Sodium	blue angels, bluebirds
pentobarbital sodium	Nembutal	nebbies, yellow bullets
phenobarbital sodium	Luminal	phennies, purple hearts
amobarbital/secobarbital	Tuinal	Christmas trees, tooies, rainbows, double-trouble
Other sedative-hypnotics		
methaqualone	Quaalude	sopors, ludes
glutethimide	Doriden	CIBA's, packs (w/codeine)
methyprylon	Noludar	
ethchlorvynol	Placidyl	
chloral hydrate	Noctec	
meprobamate	Miltown	

Central nervous system stimulants

cocaine hydrochloride	cocaine	coke, blow, toot, girl
cocaine freebase		crack, rock, base
amphetamine/ dextroamphetamine	Biphetamine T	black beauties
amphetamine sulfate	Benzedrine	A's, beans, bennies, cartwheels, hearts
amphetamine sulfate/amobarbital	Dexamyl	greenies
dextroamphetamine sulfate	Dexedrine	brownies, dexies, hearts
methamphetamine hydrochloride	Methedrine Desoxyn	bombit, crank, crystal, speed

Drugs with hallucinogenic properties

D-lysergic acid diethylamide	synthetic derivative (ergot fungus)	acid, sandos, pink wedges, sugar cubes
psilocin/psilocybin	mushroom	businessman's acid, magic mushroom
dimethyltryptamine (DMT)	synthetic	DMT, DET, DPT
morning glory seeds	bindweed (*Rivea corymbosa*)	flower power, heavenly blue, pearly gates
mescaline	peyote cactus	barf tea, big chief, mesc
methyldimethoxy- amphetamine (DOM)	synthetic (derivative)	STP

Class	Trade name(s)	Street name(s)
methylenedioxymeth-amphetamine (MDMA)	synthetic derivative	ecstacy
methylenedioxy-amphetamine (MDA)	synthetic derivative	eve
myristicin	nutmeg	MMDA
muscarine	mushroom	fly
phencyclidine		angel dust, PCP, dust
Tetrahydrocannabinoids		
marijuana	*Cannabis sativa* (leaves, flowers)	grass, hay, joints, Mary Jane, pot, reefer, rope
hashish	*Cannabis sativa* (resin)	hash
Volatile solvents and gases		
benzine	gasoline	
toluol	glue vapor	
carbon tetrachloride	cleaning fluid	
naphtha	cleaning fluid	scrubwoman's kick
amyl nitrite	amyl nitrite	amys, pears, snapper
nitrous oxide	nitrous oxide	laughing gas, nitrous

Note. Many of these drugs are sold under a variety of trade names; only a single popular example is used for each.

List of Legal Terms

best interests of the child General standard applied by courts to determine the "care and custody of minor children." Different states consider different factors relevant in defining what constitutes a "child's best interests." Some of the more common factors include the mental and physical health of all individuals involved (e.g., child, parents); the wishes of the child as to his or her choice of custodian; and the interaction and degree of "psychological connectedness" between the child and the proposed custodian.

beyond a reasonable doubt That measure or degree of proof that will produce in the mind of the trier of facts a near-certain belief or conviction as to the allegations sought to be established. Of the three legal standards of proof, this is the highest level and the one required to establish the guilt of someone accused of a crime. Sometimes thought to represent a 95 out of 100 chance of certainty. See also *clear and convincing evidence; preponderance of the evidence.*

clear and convincing evidence The second-highest level or standard applied to determining whether alleged facts have been proven. This is the standard applied to civil commitment matters and similar circumstances in which there is the chance that valued civil liberty interests and freedoms are at stake. Sometimes thought to represent a 75 out of 100 chance of certainty. See also *beyond a reasonable doubt; preponderance of the evidence.*

competency Generally refers to some minimal mental, cognitive, or behavioral ability, trait, or capability required to perform a particular legal act or to assume some legal role. See also *competency to stand trial; informed consent; testamentary capacity.*

competency to stand trial Legal test applied to all criminal defendants regarding their cognitive ability at the time of trial to participate in the proceedings against them. As held in *Dusky v. United States* (1960), a defendant is competent to stand trial if 1) he or she possesses a factual understanding of the proceedings against him or her, and 2) he or she has sufficient present ability to consult with his or her lawyer with a reasonable degree of rational understanding.

confidentiality The situation in which certain communications between persons who are in a fiduciary or trust relationship to each other (e.g., physician-patient) are generally not legally permitted to be disclosed and are not admissible as evidence in court during a trial.

conservatorship The appointment of a person to manage and make decisions on behalf of an incompetent person regarding the latter's estate (e.g., authority to make contracts or sell property). See also *guardianship.*

de facto Something that is in fact, in deed, or actually in effect. Compare with *de jure.*

de jure Something that is considered "lawful," "rightful," "legitimate," or "just." Compare with *de facto.*

diminished capacity Refers to "insufficient cognitive ability to achieve the state of mind (*mens rea*) requisite for the commission of a crime." Sometimes referred to as "partial insanity," this doctrine permits a court to consider the impaired mental state of the defendant for purposes of reducing punishment or lowering the degree of the offense being charged.

durable power of attorney A person designated by another to act as his or her attorney-in-fact regardless of whether the principal eventually becomes incompetent. This is prescribed statutorily in all 50 states. See also *living will.*

emancipated minor A person under 18 years of age who is considered totally self-supporting. Legal rights afforded at adulthood are typically extended to an emancipated minor.

expert witness One who by reason of specialized education, experience, and/or training possesses superior knowledge about a subject that is beyond the understanding of an average or ordinary layperson. Expert witnesses are permitted to offer opinions about matters relevant to their expertise that will assist the trier of facts (e.g., jury) in comprehending evidence that the trier would otherwise not understand or fully appreciate.

Gault decision A landmark Supreme Court decision in 1967 that found that juveniles were entitled to the same due process rights as adults—that is, the right to counsel, the right to notice of specific charges of the offense, the right to confront and cross-examine a witness, the right to remain silent, and the right to subpoena witnesses in defense. The right to trial by jury was not included.

guardianship The delegation, by the state, of authority over an individual's person or estate to another party. For example, a personal guardian for a mentally ill patient would have the legal right to make medical decisions on behalf of the patient.

habeas corpus (Latin, "you have the body") An order to bring a party before a judge or court; specifically, in regard to a person who is being retained within a hospital, to give the court the opportunity to examine that person and decide on the appropriateness of such retention.

informed consent In medical jurisprudence, a physician must disclose to a patient sufficient information regarding a proposed procedure to enable the patient

to make a knowing decision about whether to participate. In addition to sufficient information, any consent given must be voluntary and made by a person
considered legally competent.

insanity In law, the term denotes that degree of mental
illness that negates an individual's legal responsibility
or capacity.

insanity defense A legal concept that holds that a
person cannot be held criminally responsible for his
or her actions because, due to a mental illness, the
person was unable to form the requisite intent for
the crime he or she is charged with at the time the
crime was committed. Historically a number of standards or tests have been devised to define criminal
insanity. Some of these include the following:

> **American Law Institute/Model Penal Code test** A
> defendant would not be responsible for his or her
> criminal conduct if, as a result of mental disease or
> defect, he or she "lacked substantial capacity either
> to appreciate the criminality of his or her conduct
> or to conform his or her conduct to the require-
> ments of law."

> **Crime Control Act (CCA) of 1984 standard** In
> 1984, as part of sweeping federal legislation, the
> CCA altered the test for insanity in federal courts by
> holding that it was an affirmative defense to all
> federal crimes that at the time of the offense, "the
> defendant, as a result of a severe mental disease or
> defect, was unable to appreciate the nature and
> quality or the wrongfulness of his [or her] acts.
> Mental disease or defect does not otherwise consti-
> tute a defense."

> **Durham rule** A ruling by the U.S. Court of Appeals
> for the District of Columbia Circuit in 1954 that held
> that an accused person is not criminally responsible
> if his or her "unlawful act was the product of mental
> disease or mental defect." This decision was quite

controversial, and within several years it was modified and then replaced altogether by the same court that originally formulated it.

irresistible impulse test Acquittal of criminal responsibility is allowed if a defendant's mental disorder caused him or her to experience an "irresistible and uncontrollable impulse to commit the offense, even if he [or she] remained able to understand the nature of the offense and its wrongfulness."

M'Naughten rule In 1843, the English House of Lords ruled that a person was not responsible for a crime if the accused "was laboring under such a defect of reason from a disease of mind as not to know the nature and quality of the act; or, if he knew it, that he did not know he was doing what was wrong." This rule, or some derivation of it, is still applied in many states today.

living will Procedure by which competent persons can, under certain situations, direct their doctors to treat them in a prescribed way if they become incompetent (e.g., withdraw life-saving medical care if in a vegetative state). See also *durable power of attorney.*

medical malpractice Generally defined as "the failure to exercise the degree of skill in diagnosis or treatment that reasonably can be expected from one licensed and holding oneself out as a physician under the circumstances of a particular case." See also *negligence; standard of care; tort.*

mens rea Literally, "guilty mind." One of two fundamental aspects of any crime. The other aspect is the act, or *actus rea.*

negligence In medical malpractice law, generally described as the failure to do something that a reasonable practitioner would have done (omission) or as doing something that a reasonable practitioner would not have done (commission) under particular circumstances. See also *medical malpractice; standard of care; tort.*

preponderance of the evidence The lowest of three levels or standards applied to determining whether alleged facts have been proven. This is the standard applied to civil lawsuits. It is sometimes thought to represent a 51 out of 100 chance of certainty.

privilege A statutorily based right of the patient to restrict or bar the disclosure of confidential information in a court of law in most circumstances. See also *confidentiality.*

standard of care In the law of medical negligence, that degree of care that a reasonably prudent medical practitioner having ordinary skill, training, and learning would exercise under the same or similar circumstances. Unless the practitioner is considered an expert or specialist, the requisite degree of care is held to be only "ordinary" and "reasonable" care. If a physician's conduct falls below the standard of care, he or she may be liable in damages for any injuries resulting from such conduct.

subpoena A command, typically at the request of a litigating party, to appear at a certain time and place to give testimony on a certain matter. Unless signed by a judge, a subpoena is not a court order compelling testimony but merely a court-issued order to show up.

subpoena duces tecum A command to produce specified records or documents at a certain time and place at trial.

Tarasoff rule Based on the 1976 California decision *Tarasoff v. The Regents of the University of California,* this landmark opinion held that when a patient presents a serious danger of violence to a foreseeable victim, the psychotherapist of that patient has a duty to use reasonable care to protect the intended victim against such danger. No fewer than 30 jurisdictions have issued a ruling or statute involving some variation of the Tarasoff "duty to protect" doctrine.

testamentary capacity Pertains to the state of mind of an individual at the time he or she writes or executes his or her will. Generally, to have sufficient testamentary capacity, testators must possess a certain level of understanding of the nature and extent of their property, of the persons who are the natural objects of their bounty, and of the disposition that they are making of their property, and must appreciate these elements in relation to each other and form an orderly desire as to the disposition of their property.

tort Civil wrongs subject to lawsuit by private individuals, as distinguished from criminal offenses, which are only brought or prosecuted by the state on behalf of its citizens.

vicarious liability Indirect legal responsibility for the actions or conduct of those over whom the principal has control. For example, a private physician is generally vicariously liable for the negligence of any assisting employees.

List of Neurologic Deficits

abulia A reduction in impulse to action and thought coupled with indifference or lack of concern about the consequences of action.

acalculia Loss of previously possessed facility with arithmetic calculation.

adiadochokinesia Inability to perform rapid alternating movements of one or more of the extremities.

agnosia Inability to recognize objects presented by way of one or more sensory modalities that cannot be explained by a defect in elementary sensation or a reduced level of consciousness or alertness.

   spatial agnosia Inability to recognize spatial relations; disordered spatial orientation.

agraphia Loss of a previously possessed facility for writing.

akathisia A state of motor restlessness ranging from a feeling of inner disquiet to inability to sit still or lie quietly.

akinetic mutism A state of apparent alertness with following eye movements but no speech or voluntary motor responses.

alexia Loss of a previously possessed reading facility that cannot be explained by defective visual acuity.

anosognosia The apparent unawareness of or failure to recognize one's own functional defect (e.g., hemiplegia, hemianopsia).

aphasia Loss of a previously possessed facility of language comprehension or production that cannot be explained by sensory or motor defects or by diffuse cerebral dysfunction.

anomic or amnestic aphasia Loss of the ability to name objects.

Broca's aphasia Loss of the ability to comprehend language coupled with production of inappropriate language.

Wernicke's aphasia Loss of the ability to comprehend language coupled with production of inappropriate language.

apraxia Loss of a previously possessed ability to perform skilled motor acts that cannot be explained by weakness, abnormal muscle tone, or elementary incoordination.

constructional apraxia An acquired difficulty in drawing two-dimensional objects or forms, or in producing or copying three-dimensional arrangements of forms or shapes.

astereognosis Inability to recognize familiar objects by touch that cannot be explained by a defect of elementary tactile sensation.

ataxia Failure of muscle coordination; irregularity of muscle action.

autotopagnosia Inability to localize and name the parts of one's own body.

finger agnosia Autotopagnosia restricted to the fingers.

confabulation Fabrication of stories in response to questions about situations or events that are not recalled.

dys- Prefix usually used to indicate that a function has never developed normally: thus dyscalculia, dysgraphia, dyslexia, dysphasia, and dyspraxia. The prefix may also be used to indicate a perversion of normal function or an incomplete defect.

dysarthria Difficulty in speech production due to incoordination of the speech apparatus.

dysgeusia Perversion of the sense of taste.

echolalia Parrot-like repetition of overheard words or fragments of speech.

Gegenhalten "Active" resistance to passive movement of the extremities that does not appear to be under voluntary control.

perseveration Tendency to emit the same verbal or motor response again and again to varied stimuli.

prosopagnosia Inability to recognize familiar faces that is not explained by defective visual acuity or reduced consciousness or alertness.

sensory extinction Failure to report sensory stimuli from one region if another region is stimulated simultaneously, even though when the region in question is stimulated by itself, the stimulus is correctly reported.

simultanagnosia Inability to comprehend more than one element of a visual scene at the same time or to integrate the parts into a whole.

Table of Psychological Tests

Test	Type	What test assesses	Age of patient	Output	Admin-istration
Bayley Scales of Infant Development	Infant development	Cognitive functioning	1–30 months	Performance on subtests measuring cognitive and motor development	Individual
Bender Visual Motor Gestalt Test	Projective visual-motor development; ego function and structure; organic brain damage	Personality conflicts	5–Adult	Patient's reproduction of geometric figures	Individual

Test	Type	What test assesses	Age of patient	Output	Admin- istration
Benton Visual Retention Test	Objective performance	Organic brain damage	Adult	Patient's reproduction of geometric figures from memory	Individual
Boston Diagnostic Aphasia Exam	Clinical ratings of language performance	Aphasic disorders	Adult	Profile of deficit areas	Individual
California Verbal Learning Test	Neuropsycho- logical test of learning and memory ability	Verbal and nonverbal learning; short- and long-term memory	Adult	Multiple indices of capacity	Individual

Cattell Infant Intelligence	Infant development	General motor and cognitive development	1–18 months	Performance on developmental tasks	Individual
Child Behavior Checklist	Rating scale	Internalizing and externalizing behavior disorders	7–16	Behavior profile	Group or individual
Draw-A-Person Draw-A-Family House, Tree	Projective	Personality conflicts; self-image (DAP); family perception (DAF); ego functions; intellectual functioning (DAP); visual-motor coordination	2–Adult	Patient's drawings on a blank sheet of paper	Individual

Test	Type	What test assesses	Age of patient	Output	Admin- istration
Drug Use Screening Inventory	Self-report; paper, pencil, or computer administration	Ten domains of health, psychiatric and psycho-social severity	10–Adult	Profile of problem severity	Individual or group
Family Assessment Measure	Paper and pencil	Multiple areas and causes of family dysfunction	Children and adults	Profile of family organization and functioning	Individual or group
Frostig Developmental Test of Visual Perception	Visual perception	Eye-motor coordination; figure-ground perception; constancy of shape; position in space; spatial relationships	4–8 years	Performance on paper-and-pencil test measuring five aspects of visual perception	Individual or group

Gessell Developmental Schedules	Preschool development	Cognitive, motor, and language and social development	1–60 months	Performance on developmental tasks	Individual
Halstead-Reitan Neuropsychological Battery and Other Measures	Brain functioning	Cerebral functioning and organic brain damage	6–Adult	Various subtests measure aspects of cerebral functioning	Individual
Illinois Test of Psycholinguistic Ability (ITPA)	Language ability	Auditory-vocal, visual-motor channels of language; receptive, organizational, and expressive components	2–10 years	Performance on 12 subtests measuring various dimensions of language functioning	Individual
Luria-Nebraska Neuropsychological Battery	Cognitive and psychomotor tests	Brain integrity, lesion location	Adult and older children	Verbal and behavior responses	Individual

Test	Type	What test assesses	Age of patient	Output	Administration
Michigan Picture Stories	Defensive structure	Personality conflicts	Adolescent	Patient makes up stories after viewing stimulus pictures	Individual
Minnesota Multiphasic Personality Inventory (MMPI)	Paper and pencil; personality inventory	Personality structure; diagnostic classification	Adolescent–adult	Personality profile reflecting nine dimensions of personality; diagnosis based upon actuarial prediction	Group
Multidimensional Personality Questionnaire	Paper and pencil	Personality traits from a behavior-generic perspective	16 and older	Profile of personality characteristics	Group or individual

Raven Progressive Matrices	Self-report; paper and pencil	Nonverbal intelligence	Children and adults	Percentile rank of intelligence score	Group and individual
Rorschach	Projective	Personality conflicts, ego function and structure; defensive structure; thought processes; affective integration	3–Adult	Patient's associations to inkblots	Individual
Stanford-Binet	Intelligence	Intellectual functioning	2–Adult	Performance on problem-solving and developmental tasks	Individual

Test	Type	What test assesses	Age of patient	Output	Administration
Thematic Apperception Test (TAT)	Projective	Personality conflicts	Adult	Patient makes up stories after viewing stimulus pictures	Individual
Vineland Social Maturity Scale	Social maturity	Capacity for independent functioning	0–25+ years	Performance on developmental tasks measuring various dimensions of social functioning	Interview patient or guardian of patient, occasional self-report
Wechsler Adult Intelligence Scale (WAIS)	Intelligence	Intellectual functioning	16–Adult	Performance on 10 subtests measuring various dimensions of intellectual functioning	Individual

Wechsler Intelligence Scale for Children (WISC)	Intelligence	Intellectual functioning; thought processes; ego functioning	5–15	Performance on 10 subtests measuring various dimensions of intellectual functioning	Individual
Wechsler Memory Scale	Psychiatric examination of memory ability	Verbal and nonverbal memory	Adult	Memory quotient and scores quantifying different aspects of memory capacity	Individual
Wechsler Preschool Primary Scale of Intelligence (WPPSI)	Intelligence	Intellectual functioning; thought processes; ego functioning	4–6½ years	Performance on 10 subtests measuring various dimensions of intellectual functioning	Individual

Test	Type	What test assesses	Age of patient	Output	Admin-istration
Wisconsin Card Sort	Neuropsycho-logical test of card sorting to defined concept	Abstracting ability, especially sensitive to anterior frontal lobes	Adult	Concept learning ability measures of cognitive flexibility	Individual

List of Research Terms

analysis of variance (ANOVA) A widely used statistical procedure for determining the significance of differences obtained on an experimental variable studied under two or more conditions. Differences are commonly assigned to three aspects: the individual differences among the subjects or patients studied; group differences, however classified (e.g., by sex); and differences according to the various treatments to which the subjects have been assigned. The method can assess both the main effects of a variable and its interaction with other variables that have been studied simultaneously.

attributable risk The rate of the disorder in exposed subjects that can be attributed to the exposure; derived from subtracting the rate (usually incidence or mortality) of the disorder of the nonexposed population from the corresponding rate of the exposed population.

concordance In genetic studies, the similarity in a twin pair with respect to the presence or absence of a disease or trait.

control The term is used in three contexts: 1) keeping the relevant conditions of an experiment constant, 2) causing an *independent variable* to vary in a specified and known manner, and 3) using a spontaneously occurring and discoverable fact as a check or standard of comparison to evaluate the facts obtained after the manipulation of the independent variable.

control group In the ideal case, a group of subjects matched as closely as possible to an experimental group of subjects on all relevant aspects and exposed to the same treatments except the independent variable under investigation.

correlation The extent to which two measures vary together, or a measure of the strength of the relationship between two variables. It is usually expressed by a coefficient that varies between +1.0 (perfect agreement) and −1.0 (a perfect inverse relationship). A correlation coefficient of 0.0 would mean a perfectly random relationship. The correlation coefficient signifies the degree to which knowledge of one score or variable can predict the score on the other variable. A high correlation between two variables does not necessarily indicate a causal relationship between them; the correlation may follow because each of the variables is highly related to a third, as yet unmeasured, factor.

criterion variable Something to be predicted.

demand characteristics The sum total of cues that communicates the purpose of the experiment and the nature of the behavior expected of the subject. (The cues are derived from the manner in which the subject is solicited, the manner in which he or she is treated by the experimenter, the scuttlebutt about the experiment, the experimental instructions, and, most important, the experimental procedure itself.) Subjects may confirm the investigator's hypothesis in an effort to behave appropriately rather than respond directly to the independent variables under investigation. By extension, as applied to nonexperimental settings, the tendency of individuals to live up to what is implicitly expected of them, a factor that may play a major role in the outcome of treatment.

discordance In genetic studies, dissimilarity in a twin pair with respect to the presence or absence of a disease or trait.

double-blind Referring to a study design in which a number of treatments, usually one or more drugs and a placebo, are compared in such a way that neither the patient nor the persons directly involved in the treatment know which preparation is being administered.

ecological validity The extent to which controlled experimental results can be generalized beyond the confines of the particular experimental context of a variety of contexts in the real world.

experimental design The logical framework of an experiment that maximizes the probability of obtaining or detecting real effects and minimizes the likelihood of ambiguities regarding the significance of the experimentally observed differences.

experimental study designs

    case control An investigation in which groups of individuals are selected in terms of whether they do (cases) or do not (controls) have the disorder the etiology of which is being studied.

    cohort An important form of epidemiological investigation to test hypotheses regarding the causation of disease. The distinguishing factors are that 1) the group or groups of persons to be studied (the cohorts) are defined in terms of characteristics evident prior to appearance of the disorder being investigated; and 2) the study groups so defined are observed over a period of time to determine the frequency of the disorder among them.

    cross-sectional Study in which measurements are made in different samples at the same point in time.

    independent group Study in which different treatments are given to different groups; for example, comparing an untreated group with a treated group. Methodologically very sound, but often requires large samples if there is much variability between individuals.

    longitudinal Study in which observations on the same individuals are made at two or more different points in time. Most cohort and case-control studies are longitudinal.

prospective Study based on data or events that occur subsequent in time relative to the initiation of the investigation. This type of predictive study usually requires many years in order to develop a large enough study population.

retrospective Study based on data or events that occurred prior in time relative to the investigation.

subjects as their own control The same individual is compared with herself or himself before and after a given treatment. This has the advantage of decreasing error variance and the likelihood of showing significant differences with relatively small groups, though it has the disadvantage of practice effects that may occur with repeated measurements.

experimenter bias Experimenter expectations that are inadvertently communicated to patients or subjects. Such expectations may influence experimental findings.

external validity The applicability of the generalizations that may be made from the experimental findings beyond the occasion with those specific subjects, experimental conditions, experimenters, or measurements.

falsifiable hypothesis A hypothesis stated in sufficiently precise fashion that it can be tested by acceptable rules of logic and empirical and statistical evidence, and thereby found to be either confirmed or disconfirmed. An unfalsifiable hypothesis is one that is so general and/or ambiguous that all conceivable evidence can be "explained" by it.

heuristic Serving to encourage discovery of problem solutions.

incidence The number of cases of disease that come into being during a specific period of time.

intervening variable Something intervening between an antecedent circumstance and its consequence, modifying the relation between the two. For example, appetite can be an intervening variable determining whether or not a given food will be eaten. The intervening variable may be inferred rather than empirically detected.

mean The arithmetic average of a set of observations; the sum of scores divided by the number of scores.

median The middle value in a set of values that have been arranged in order from highest to lowest.

mode The most frequently occurring observation in a set of observations.

nonparametric tests of significance Specialized statistical procedures that do not require assumptions of normality when data do not satisfy certain statistical assumptions, such as being normally distributed. These procedures are often based on an analysis of ranks rather than on the distribution of the actual scores themselves. Widely used examples are the chi-square, Spearman rank order correlation, median, and Mann-Whitney U tests.

null hypothesis Predicting that an experiment will show no difference between conditions or no relationship between variables. Statistical tests are then applied to the results of the experiment to try to disprove the null hypothesis. Testing requires a computation to determine the limits within which two groups may differ in their results (e.g., an experimental and a control group) even though if the experiment were often repeated or the groups were larger no difference would be found. The probability of the obtained difference being found if no true difference existed is commonly expressed as a P value (e.g., P less than .05 that the null hypothesis is true).

operational definition The meaning of a concept when it is translated to terms amenable to systematic observation and measurement (e.g., temperature defined by a thermometer reading under standard conditions).

parameter Any quantitative value that a variable can take.

parametric study One that examines the effects on a dependent variable of variations, usually across a broad range, in the base values of the independent variable.

parametric tests of significance Tests based on the assumption that the form of the distribution of the observations is known, usually a so-called normal distribution. Widely used tests based on such an assumption include analysis of variance, t tests, and Pearson coefficient of correlation.

period prevalence A measure that expresses the total number of cases of a disease known to have existed at some time during a specified period. It is the sum of point prevalence and incidence.

placebo In psychopharmacology, a pill that contains no pharmacologically active ingredient.

> **active placebo** A placebo that may mimic the side effects but does not have the specific and assumed therapeutic pharmacological action of the drug under investigation.

> **placebo effect** Either therapeutic effects or side effects following the ingestion of a placebo. By extension, one may speak of a placebo effect as comprising the nonspecific aspects of any treatment procedure, usually mediated by the patient's expectations of improvement, such as the placebo effect of psychotherapy.

point prevalence The frequency of the disease at a designated point in time.

population A statistical concept that refers to all individuals or instances that theoretically could be available for study or measurement. Statistical inference involves generalizing from the observation of some specified sample to the population.

practice effects The modification in task performances as a result of repeated trials or training in the task.

predictor variable The test or other form of performance that is used to predict the person's status on a criterion variable. For example, scores on the Scholastic Aptitude Test might be used to predict the criterion "finishing college within the top 33% of graduating class." Scores on the SAT would be predictor scores.

quantitative variable An object of observation that varies in manner or degree in such a way that it may be measured.

Q-sort A personality assessment technique in which the subject (or some observer) indicates the degree to which a standardized set of descriptive statements actually describes him or her (the subject). The term reflects the "sorting" procedures occasionally used with this technique.

random sample A group of subjects selected in such a way that each member of the population from which the sample is derived has an equal or known chance (i.e., probability) of being chosen for the sample.

relative risk The ratio of the disorder (usually incidence of mortality) of those exposed to the disorder to the rate of those not exposed.

reliability The extent to which the same test or procedure will yield the same result either over time or with different observers. The most commonly reported reliabilities are as follows:

test-retest reliability The correlation between the first and second test of a number of subjects.

split-half reliability The correlation within a single test of two similar parts of the test.

interrater reliability The agreement between different individuals scoring the same procedure or observations.

selection bias The inadvertent selection of a nonrep-
resentative sample of subjects or observations. A
classic example is a 1936 *Literary Digest* poll that
predicted Landon's election over Roosevelt in which
telephone directories were used as the basis for
selecting respondents.

significance level The arbitrarily selected probability
level for rejecting the null hypothesis, commonly 0.05
or 0.01.

significant differences Statistical tests showing that a
given difference is not likely to have occurred by
chance. In many behavioral studies, the likelihood of
an event occurring less frequently than 1 in 20 times
($P < 0.05$) is considered the minimal acceptable significance level. The determination that a given difference
between two groups is significant can merely serve to
identify the likelihood that it was not a chance event.
In no way does this prove that the demonstrated
systematic difference is necessarily due to the reasons
hypothesized by an investigator. Systematic factors not
considered by the investigator can sometimes be
responsible for significant differences.

standard deviation (SD) A mathematical measure of
the dispersion or spread of scores clustered about the
mean. In any distribution that approximates the normal curve in form, about 65% of the measurements
will lie within one SD of the mean, and about 95% will
lie within two SDs of the mean.

statistical inference The process of using a limited
sample of data to infer something about a larger
population of potentially obtainable data that have not
been observed.

test of significance A comparison of the observed
probability of an event with the predicted probability
that is based on calculations deduced from statistical
chance distributions of such events.

theory A general statement predicting, explaining, or describing the relationships among a number of constructs.

type I error The error that is made when the null hypothesis is true but, as the result of the test of significance, is rejected or declared false.

type II error The error that is made when the null hypothesis is false but, as a result of the test of significance, is not rejected or declared false.

variable Any characteristic in an experiment that may assume different values.

    independent variable The variable under the experimenter's control.

    dependent variable That aspect of the subject that is measured after the manipulation of the independent variable and that is assumed to vary as a function of the independent variable.

variance The square of the standard deviation.

volunteer bias Bias that may occur when individuals who volunteer for some procedures are not generally representative of the total population. Self-selected patients who seek out treatment based on newspaper publicity, for example, are likely to do significantly better than random patients who are simply offered the treatment.

zygosity 1) Dizygotic: fraternal twins, the product of two fertilized ova. They have the genetic relationship of any two siblings. 2) Monozygotic: identical twins, the product of a single fertilized ovum.

Outline of Schools of Psychiatry

I. Reconstructive

   A. Psychoanalysis—Sigmund Freud

   B. Neo-Freudian, modifications of psychoanalysis
1. Active analytic techniques—Sandor Ferenczi, Wilhelm Stekel, the Chicago school (especially Franz Alexander and Thomas French)
2. Analytic play therapy—Anna Freud, Melanie Klein
3. Analytic psychology—Carl Jung
4. Character analysis, orgone therapy— Wilhelm Reich
5. Cognitive—Jean Piaget
6. Developmental—Erik Erikson
7. Ego psychology—Paul Federn, Edoardo Weiss, Heinz Hartmann, Ernst Kris, Rudolph Loewenstein
8. Object relations—Melanie Klein, W. R. D. Fairbairn, D. W. Winnicott, Otto Kernberg, Margaret Mahler, Edith Jacobson
9. Self psychology—Heinz Kohut
10. Existential analysis—Ludwig Binswanger
11. Holistic analysis—Karen Horney
12. Individual psychology—Alfred Adler
13. Transactional analysis—Eric Berne

14. Washington cultural school—Harry Stack Sullivan, Erich Fromm, Clara Thompson
15. Will therapy—Otto Rank

C. Group Approaches

1. Orthodox psychoanalytic—S. R. Slavson
2. Psychodrama—J. L. Moreno
3. Psychoanalysis in groups—Alexander Wolf
4. Valence systems—W. R. Bion

II. Reeducative and Supportive, Individual and Group

A. Client-centered (nondirective)—Carl Rogers

B. Conditioning, behavior therapy, behavior modification

1. Aversion therapy—N. V. Kantorovich
2. Behaviorism—John B. Watson
3. Classical conditioning—Ivan Pavlov
4. Operant conditioning—B. F. Skinner
5. Sexual counseling—William Masters, Virginia Johnson
6. Systematic desensitization—Joseph Wolpe

C. Cognitive-behavior therapy—Aaron Beck

D. Family therapy—Nathan Ackerman

E. Gestalt—Wolfgang Köhler, Kurt Lewin, Fritz Perls

F. Logotherapy—Viktor Frankl

G. Psychobiology (distributive analysis and synthesis)—Adolf Meyer

H. Zen (satori)—Alan Watts